INTERPRETING ECGs

An advanced self-test guide

Second Edition

Ali Haddad, MD   David C. Dean, MD

Medical Economics Book
Oradell, N.J. 07649

D0813889

Acquisitions Editor: Thomas Bentz
Production Editor: Dorothy Erstling
Cover Design: Brianne Carey Wright
Design: James M. Walsh
Original Art: Janet Kroenke
Art Director: Sharyn Banks
Typesetting: Text Processing

Library of Congress Cataloging in Publication Data

Haddad, Ali
  Interpreting ECGs.

  Includes index.
  1. Electrocardiography—Case studies. 1.   Dean,
David C. II. Title. [DNLM: 1. Electrocardiography—
Examination questions.   WG18 H126i]
RC683.5.ESH25   616.1'207547'076   80-15313
ISBN 0-87489-447-6

Medical Economics Company Inc.
Oradell, New Jersey 07649

Printed in the United States of America

616.12075470 76
H126,
1987

CONTENTS

Publisher's Notes
Preface
Commonly Used Abbreviations
Section I   **TABLES**   *1*
Section II   **SINUS AND SUPRAVENTRICULAR ARRHYTHMIAS**   *9*
Section III   **VENTRICULAR ARRHYTHMIAS**   *65*
Section IV   **DISORDERS OF CONDUCTION**   *117*
Section V   **ATRIAL AND VENTRICULAR HYPERTROPHY**   *195*
Section VI   **MYOCARDIAL INFARCTIONS AND ISCHEMIA**   *205*
Section VII   **SPECIAL PATTERNS**   *219*
Index   *249*

PUBLISHER'S NOTES

Ali Haddad, MD, FACP, is consultant and lecturer in cardiology at Aleppo University School of Medicine in Aleppo, Syria. He received cardiology training at the State University of New York at Buffalo School of Medicine, Buffalo Veterans Administration Hospital Program between 1975 and 1977. He subsequently was a staff physician at the Iron Mountain Veterans Administration Hospital in Michigan.

David C. Dean, MD, FACP, FACC, FCCP, is chief of cardiac rehabilitation at the Buffalo Veterans Administration Medical Center, where he served as chief of the cardiopulmonary laboratory for 14 years. He is also clinical professor of medicine at the State University of New York at Buffalo, and associate physician at the Buffalo General Hospital. Dr. Dean received postgraduate training at Strong Memorial Hospital, Rochester, New York, and cardiology training at the West Roxbury Veterans Administration Hospital and the Massachusetts General Hospital in Boston.

PREFACE

The ECG strips in this book were collected from the VA Hospital of Buffalo, the VA Hospital of Iron Mountain, Michigan, Aleppo University Hospital, and the Cardio-vascular Clinic of Aleppo-Syria.

Unless otherwise mentioned, these strips are taken with a speed of 25 mm/second and full standardization. For most of the strips, we have indicated the lead used in the upper left corner. The MO (monitor) lead is halfway between V1 and V2. L1, L2, and L3 refer to limb leads.

We begin with a table of heart rates of basic cardiac arrhythmias to help in differential diagnosis, especially of atrial and junctional arrhythmias. Also included is a simple and accurate method for determining axis.

This expanded second edition with 68 new strips and revised, comprehensive section breakdowns is a small atlas of electrocardiographic abnormalities. The added strips show heart chamber hypertrophy, myocardial infarctions, bundle branch blocks, and special important cases. A few repeated arrhythmias were deleted; a few were added. Three new tables help to determine the site of a myocardial infarction.

We hope that this self-assessment tool proves useful to students, residents, and teachers of medicine.

Ali Haddad, MD
David C. Dean, MD

COMMONLY USED ABBREVIATIONS

AF: atrial fibrillation
AMI: anterior myocardial infarction
ALMI: anterolateral myocardial infarction
ASMI: anteroseptal myocardial infarction
AV: atrioventricular
CSP: carotid sinus pressure
DS: double standard
ECG/EKG: electrocardiogram
f wave: fibrillation wave
F wave: flutter wave
ILBBB: incomplete left bundle branch block
IMI: inferior myocardial infarction
IPMI: inferior posterior myocardial infarction
IRBBB: incomplete right bundle branch block
LAD: left axis deviation
LAE: left atrial enlargement
LAH: left anterior hemiblock
LBBB: left bundle branch block

LGL: Lown-Ganong-Levine
LVH: left ventricular hypertrophy
MO: monitor lead
NSR: normal sinus rhythm
PAC: premature atrial complex
PAT: paroxysmal atrial tachycardia
PMI: posterior myocardial infarction
PVC: premature ventricular complex
RAD: right axis deviation
RAE: right atrial enlargement
RBBB: right bundle branch block
RVH: right ventricular hypertrophy
SA: sinoatrial
SB: sinus bradycardia
SSS: sick sinus syndrome
ST: sinus tachycardia
st: standardization (1 millivolt)
VF: ventricular fibrillation
VT: ventricular tachycardia
WPW: Wolff-Parkinson-White

SECTION I

TABLES

Table 1

DETERMINING HEART RATE

LARGE SQUARES:			1					2					3				
SMALL SQUARES:	3	4	5	6	7	8	9	10	11	12	13	14	15	16	17	18	19
RATE:	500	375	300	250	214	187	167	150	136	125	115	107	100	94	88	83	79

LARGE SQUARES:	4					5				6					7		
SMALL SQUARES:	20	21	22	23	24	25	26	27	28	29	30	31	32	33	34	35	36
RATE:	75	71	68	65	62	60	58	56	54	52	50	48	47	45	44	43	42

LARGE SQUARES:				8					9					10			
SMALL SQUARES:	37	38	39	40	41	42	43	44	45	46	47	48	49	50	51	52	53
RATE:	41	40	39	38	37	36	35	34	33	33	32	31	31	30	30	29	28

Count the number of small or large squares between two consecutive R or P waves and use this table to determine the precise heart rate (beats per minute), provided the cardiac rhythm is regular. If this table is not available, the heart rate per minute (60 seconds) can be determined by dividing the number of large squares (each $1/5$ second) into 300 (5 × 60) or the number of small squares ($1/25$ second) into 1500 (25 × 60).

Table 2

DETERMINING AXIS

Isoelectric Lead	Reference Lead	Axis
I	AVF ↑ ↓	+ 90* − 90
II	AVF ↑ ↓	+ 150 − 30*
III	AVF ↑ ↓	+ 30* − 150
AVR	AVF ↑ ↓	+ 120 − 60*
AVL	AVF ↑ ↓	+ 60* − 120
AVF	I ↑ ↓	0* ± 180

*Most common axis for each isoelectric lead.

To determine QRS axis, find the lead in the frontal plane (leads I through AVF) that is most isoelectric where the positive voltage of the R wave is similar to the negative voltage of the Q or S wave. The QRS axis is 90° perpendicular to this lead when you consult the hexaxial reference system (Figure 1). You must look at another lead to determine if the axis is positive (+) or negative (−). AVF is an excellent reference lead except when it is the isoelectric lead. For example, if lead I is isoelectric, then the QRS axis is either +90° or −90°: if the QRS is positive (↑) in lead AVF, then the axis is +90°; if the QRS is negative (↓), then the axis is −90°.

Figure 1
THE HEXAXIAL REFERENCE SYSTEM

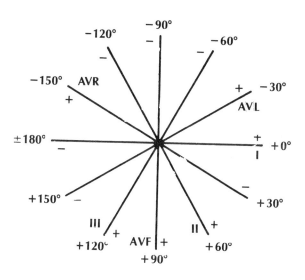

Table 3

DETERMINING THE SITE OF THE MYOCARDIAL INFARCTION: TYPE I*

The site of M.I.	The leads showing the evolutionary changes.
Anterior M.I.	V2 and V4.
Anterolateral M.I.	I, AVL, V4, V5 and V6.
Anteroseptal M.I.	V1, V2, V3 and V4.
Extensive anterior M.I.	I, AVL, V1, V2, V3, V4, V5 and V6.
Anteroinferior or apical M.I.	II, III, AVF and one or more of leads V1 to V4.
Septal M.I.	V1 and V2.
Lateral M.I.	I, AVL, V5 and V6.
High lateral M.I.	I, AVL.
Inferior M.I.	II, III and AVF.

*M.I.'s which give the standard ST-T-Q evolutionary changes.

Table 4

DETERMINING THE SITE OF THE MYOCARDIAL INFARCTION: TYPE II*

The site of the M.I.	The leads and the M.I.'s markers
Posterior M.I.	Prominent R in V1, V2 and V3.
Posteroinferior M.I.	Prominent R in V1, V2 and V3 plus the standard evolutionary changes in II, III and AVF.
Suspected subendo-cardial M.I.	1—ST depression in lead I, II, AVL and V2 to V6 for more than one week with clinical evidence of infarction and/or
	2—T wave inversion with amplitude greater than 5 mm in lead V1, V2 and V3 and to a lesser degree in V4, V5 and V6.
Suspected right ven-tricular M.I.	The standard evolutionary changes of inferior infarction plus ST elevation in lead V4R.
Suspected atrial M.I.	1—Atrial arrhythmias during the acute phase of M.I.
	2—An unusual P wave configuration.
	3—Depression or elevation of PR segment.

*M.I.'s which give unusual markers.

Table 5

HEART RATES OF BASIC ARRHYTHMIAS

Rhythm	Atrial rate	Ventricular rate
Sinus rhythm	60-100	60-100
Sinus bradycardia	45-60 (35-60)*	45-60 (35-60)
Sinus tachycardia	100-160 (100-180)	100-160 (100-180)
Sinus arrhythmia	60-100	60-100
Wandering pacemaker	60-100	60-100
Multifocal atrial tachycardia	100-200 (100-250)	100-150 (60-150)
Atrial tachycardia†	160-200 (140-300)	160-180 (140-200)
Atrial flutter	270-330 (200-400)	150-180 (120-250)
Atrial fibrillation	350-550	50-200
Junctional rhythm**		40-60
Accelerated junctional rhythm		60-100
Junctional tachycardia		100-220
Ventricular parasystole		20-60
Idioventricular rhythm		30-40 (15-40)
Accelerated idioventricular rhythm		40-100
Ventricular tachycardia		140-180 (100-250)
Torsades de Pointes		200-250
Ventricular flutter		180-250 (130-300)
Ventricular fibrillation		150-500

*The numbers in parentheses denote less common rate ranges.
**Many textbooks use the term *nodal* instead of *junctional*.
†Some textbooks use the term supraventricular tachycardia (S.V.T.) to cover both atrial tachycardia and juctional tachycardia.

SECTION II

SINUS AND SUPRAVENTRICULAR ARRHYTHMIAS

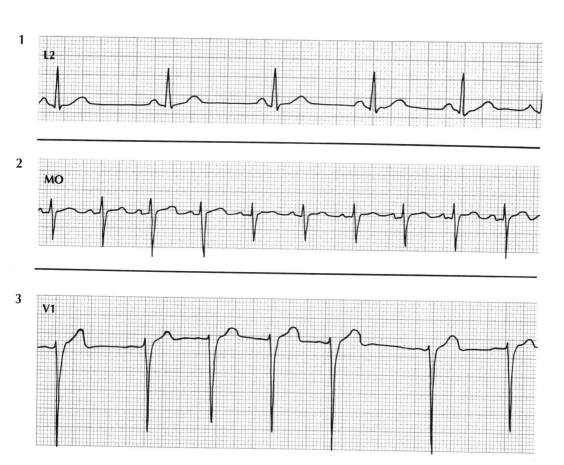

1 L2

2 MO

3 V1

1 Sinus Arrhythmia:

The heart rate changes gradually. It increases with inspiration and decreases with expiration. This is a normal and harmless phenomenon.

2 Respiratory Rhythmic Variation:

The QRS magnitude increases with expiration and decreases with inspiration, depending on the amount of lung tissue between the heart and the monitoring electrode. This is a normal finding.

3 Sinus Arrhythmia:

Both the heart rate and the QRS magnitude change with each respiratory cycle.

4

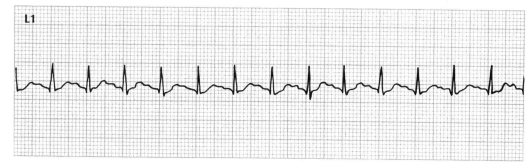

5

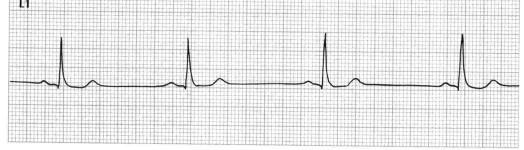

4 Sinus Tachycardia:

Every QRS complex is preceded by a P wave. The heart rate is 150/minute. In every case of sinus tachycardia with heart rate of 125 or more, atrial flutter with 2:1 block should be ruled out.

5 Sinus Bradycardia with Sinus Arrhythmia:

The rate is about 40.

Carotid sinus pressure

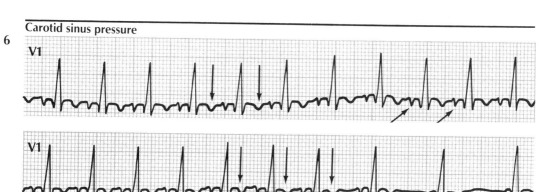

6 Sinus Tachycardia:

The upper arrows ($\downarrow$) denote T waves and the lower arrows ($\rightarrow$) denote P waves. The R wave is prominent because of RVH. Carotid sinus pressure was applied and establishes the fact that there is one P wave for each QRS complex. The heart rate slows from 120 to 72. The configuration of the P wave after carotid sinus pressure is different, suggesting that an ectopic atrial focus near the SA node is operative after the carotid sinus pressure.

7

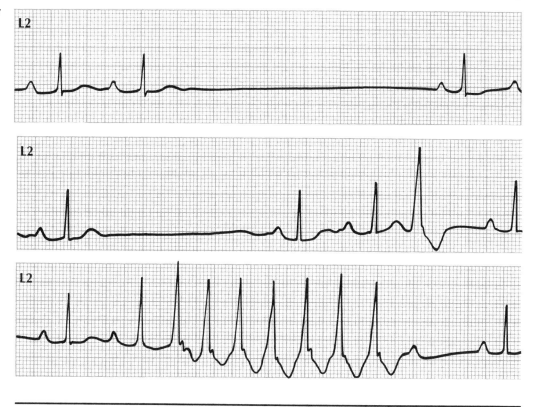

7 Bradycardia-Tachycardia Syndrome:

The basic rhythm is sinus with first degree AV block. The upper strip shows sinus arrest of 3.5 seconds. The middle strip shows sinus arrest of 2.5 seconds and one PVC. The lower strip shows a run of ventricular tachycardia at heart rate 167. The bradycardia-tachycardia syndrome is a form of sick sinus syndrome (SSS) with paroxysms of an ectopic atrial tachyarrhythmia alternating with sinus and junctional node inertia.*

*This case is unusual as ventricular tachycardia is rarely seen in this syndrome. This patient would be helped by implantation of a permanent pacemaker.

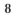

8

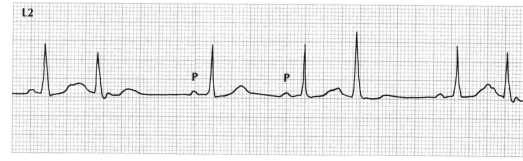

9

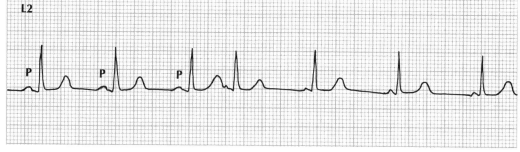

8 Premature Atrial Complexes

The second, fifth, and seventh QRS complexes are premature, and each is preceded by a P wave that changes the configuration of the preceding T wave. The second and seventh complexes also show aberrant conduction, as an S wave is now apparent. The two P waves marked P represent the basic regular PP cycle.

9 Atrial Escape:

The first three complexes are of sinus origin (P). The fourth one is a PAC. The P waves of three complexes following the PAC differ in configuration from those of the sinus complexes. The rate also slows. These complexes are called atrial escape, although some authors believe they might be due to aberrant atrial conduction.

During Valsalva maneuver

L2

10

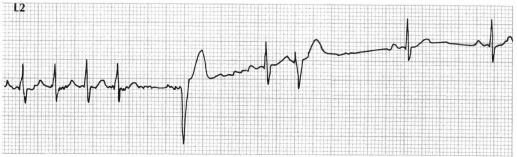

During carotid massage

11

L2

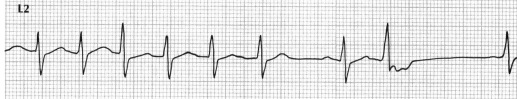

10   Supraventricular Tachycardia:

Conversion of supraventricular tachycardia at heart rate 177 to sinus rhythm by Valsalva maneuver. Note the ventricular escape beat after the termination of the arrhythmia due to vagal stimulation of the SA node.

11   Paroxysmal Atrial Tachycardia:

This PAT with heart rate 130 is converted by carotid massage to sinus rhythm. This rhythm might be mistaken for sinus tachycardia because of its slow rate, but its conversion to sinus rhythm by carotid massage is strong evidence that is it PAT.

12

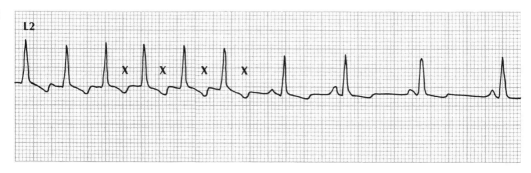

13

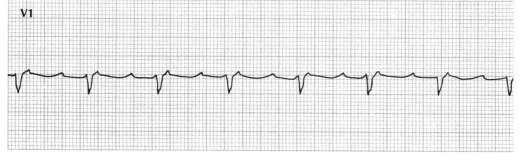

12 Atrial Tachycardia:

This first six QRS complexes form a paroxysmal atrial tachycardia with heart rate of 140. First degree AV block is present (PR .24). The P waves deform the preceding T waves (X). The rhythm converts to sinus spontaneously. Note the different T configuration with sinus rhythm.

13 Atrial Tachycardia with 2:1 AV Block:

The atrial rate is 160, and the ventricular rate is 80. The nonconducted P wave deforms the ST segment, and the conducted P wave has a prolonged PR interval of .28 second.

14

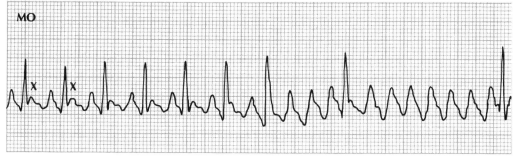

During carotid massage

15

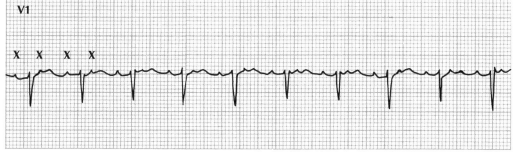

14 Atrial Tachycardia with 2:1 AV Block:

The atrial rate is 210, and the ventricular rate is 105. The first four P waves are marked X. This rhythm strip may appear to resemble sinus tachycardia if the blocked P waves are not noticed.

15 Atrial Flutter

Effect of carotid massage on atrial flutter with 2:1 AV conduction. The atrial rate is 270, and the ventricular rate is 135. The carotid massage slows the ventricular rate and the flutter waves become more apparent. This rhythm strip may appear to resemble sinus tachycardia if the nonconducted flutter waves (X) are not noticed.

16

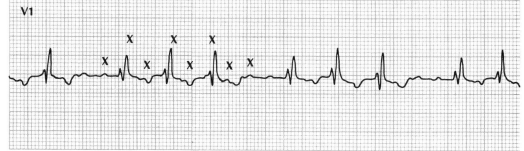

17

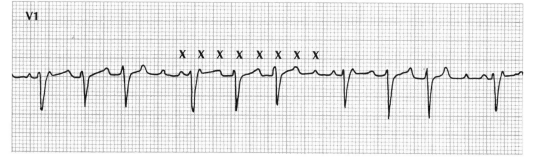

16 Atrial Flutter with Wenckebach AV Block (8:3) and Trigeminal Rhythm:

The atrial rate of 175 is within the range of atrial flutter. The flutter waves are marked X. The conducted flutter waves (first, third, and fifth) show gradual prolongation of the FR interval. The second, fourth, sixth, seventh, and eighth flutter waves are blocked. The RR interval becomes shorter as the FR interval becomes longer. Right bundle branch block is present. The first complex in each trigeminy has some aberration.

17 Atrial Flutter with Wenckebach AV Block (8:3):

The atrial rate is 300. The second, fourth, sixth, seventh, and eighth flutter waves (X) are blocked. The conducted flutter waves (first, third, and fifth) show lengthening of the FR interval. The RR interval shortens as the FR interval lengthens.

18

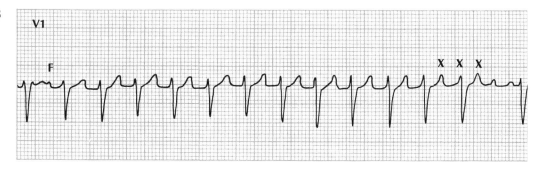

19

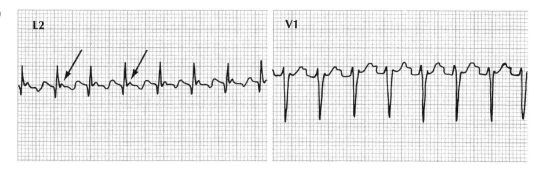

18 Atrial Flutter with 2:1 AV Block:

The atrial rate is 320, and the ventricular rate is 160. AV block increases (first X) with slight slowing of the ventricular rate. The flutter wave lost in the QRS complex becomes more apparent (second X). Concealed conduction of the AV node (third X) now prevents continuation of the 2:1 block.

19 Atrial Flutter with 2:1 AV Block:

The atrial rate is 330, and the ventricular rate is 165. Lead 2 shows the characteristic saw-toothed configuration. This rhythm strip could be confused with sinus or atrial tachycardia if the blocked flutter waves (arrows) are not noticed.

20

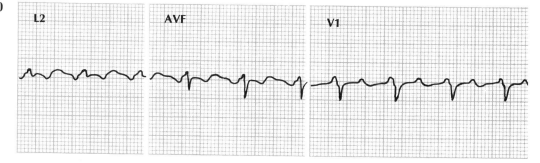

21

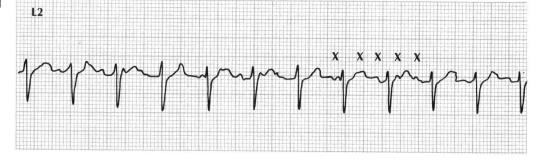

20 Atrial Flutter with 2:1 AV Block:

The atrial rate is 200, with a saw-toothed configuration in leads 2 and AVF. The ventricular rate is 100. It is unusual for the atrial rate in atrial flutter to be less than 250 unless the patient is taking quinidine, which slows the atrial rate.

21 Atrial Flutter with Junctional Tachycardia and Complete AV Dissociation:

The atrial rate is 275, and the ventricular rate is 125. There are no conducted flutter waves (X). This double tachycardia is very suggestive of digitalis toxicity.

22

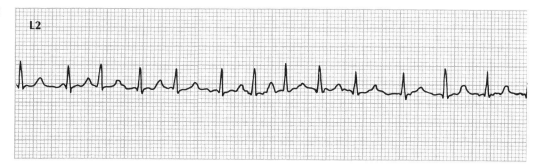

L2

22 Atrial Fibrillation:

The rhythm is irregularly irregular. There are no regularly occurring P waves. The f wave may occasionally resemble a P wave. The ventricular rate is 144 if derived by counting the QRS complexes in a five-second interval and multiplying by 12.

23

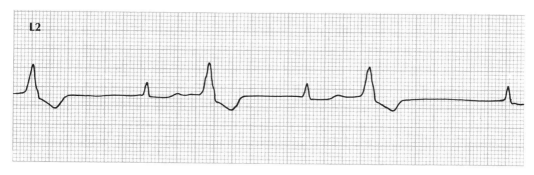

24

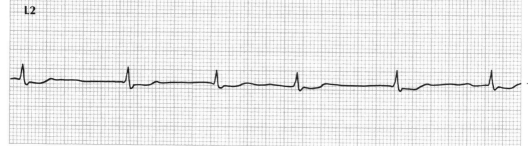

Strips 23 and 24 are from the same patient.

23 Atrial Fibrillation With Ventricular Bigeminy:

The first, third, and fifth QRS complexes are PVCs. These QRS complexes are bizarre, wide, and have fixed coupling intervals with the preceding complexes. The f waves are not seen in lead 2.

24 Fine Atrial Fibrillation:

Same patient as strip 23. The f waves are not seen in lead 2.

25

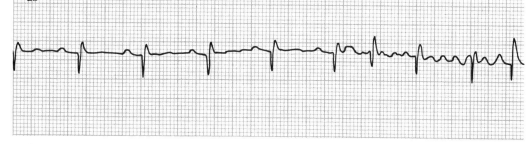

26

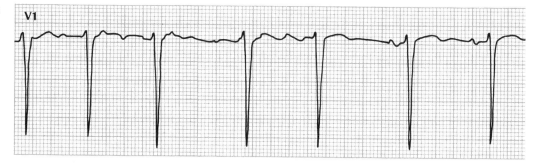

25 Conversion of Sinus Rhythm to Atrial Fibrillation:

The seventh complex is a PAC initiating an irregularly irregular rhythm with an atrial rate of about 500.

26 Conversion of Atrial Fibrillation to Sinus Rhythm:

The last two complexes are each preceded by a P wave of sinus origin, while the initial five complexes are preceded by f waves.

27

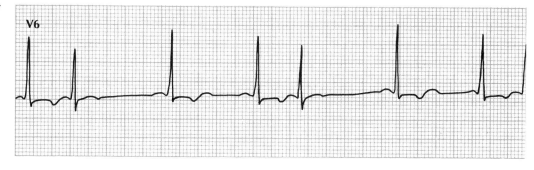

V6

28

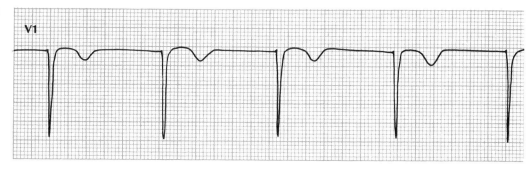

V1

27 Junctional Premature Complexes:

The second, fifth, and eighth complexes are premature and are not associated with any atrial activity.

28 Junctional Rhythm:

The ventricular rate is 50 and regular. No P waves are seen. The QRS duration is less than .12 second.

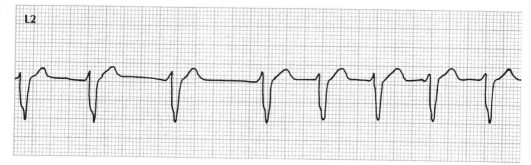

L2

29 Atrial Fibrillation and Accelerated Junctional Rhythm:

The first three RR intervals are irregular and suggest atrial fibrillation, although no f waves are seen in lead 2. The last four RR cycles are regular at heart rate of 98. No P waves are seen. This suggests a midnodal accelerated junctional rhythm. Note also that the QRS duration is wide (.12) because of an associated bundle branch block.

30

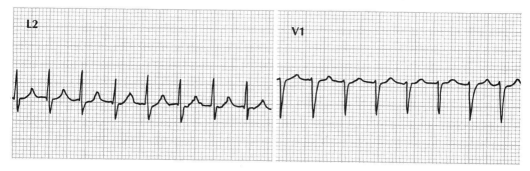

31

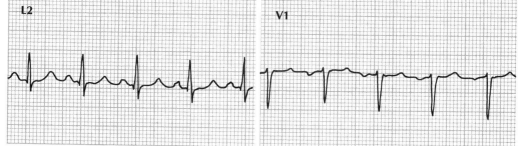

Strips 30 and 31 are from the same patient.

30 Junctional Tachycardia (Midnodal):

P waves are absent and appear to be buried in the QRS complexes. The ventricular rate is 170.

31 Sinus Tachycardia:

Same patient as strip 30. The heart rate is 102.

32

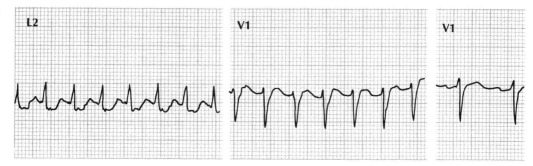

33

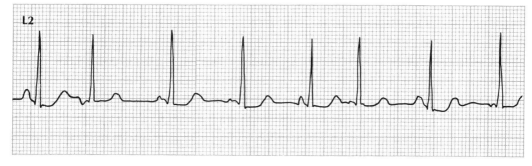

32 Supraventricular Tachycardia:

This arrhythmia is most likely junctional tachycardia. The heart rate is 190. P waves are seen following the QRS complexes in the first strip, and before the QRSs in the third strip, when conversion to sinus rhythm at heart rate 98 is noted.

33 Wandering Pacemaker:

The pacemaker wanders between the sinus node, junctional tissue, and various locations in the atrium. The first P wave is of sinus origin, the second P wave is of junctional origin, and the remainder of the P waves are of multifocal atrial origin. At least three different P wave configurations are needed in one lead to make this diagnosis.

34

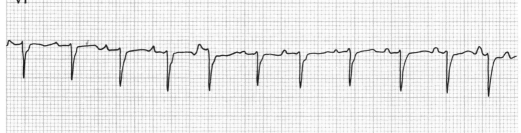

35

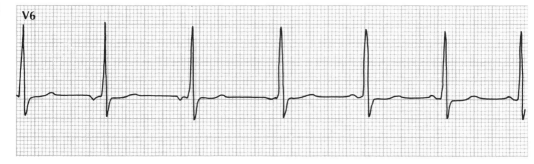

34 Multifocal Atrial Tachycardia:

The rhythm is irregular, and the P wave configuration differs significantly from beat to beat. The heart rate is 120 if derived by counting the QRS complexes for five seconds and multiplying by 12. If the heart rate were less than 100, this would be called wandering pacemaker.

35 Wandering Pacemaker:

The pacemaker wanders between junctional tissue and sinus node. The first four P waves are inverted and originate in junctional tissue. The last three P waves are upright and originate in the SA node.

36

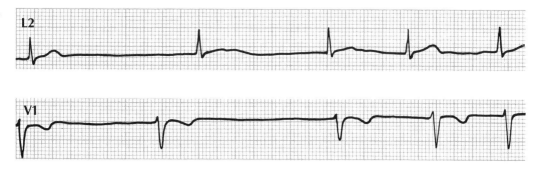

37

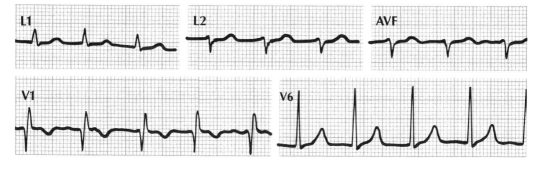

36 Atrial Fibrillation:

There is no evidence of f waves or P waves. The rhythm is irregularly irregular. This is called fine atrial fibrillation. The tracing is from a 17 year old man without evidence of heart disease.

37 Atrial Fibrillation:

The rhythm appears regular and may be mistaken for junctional or even sinus rhythm. The pseudo P waves seen in lead V1 are not a consistent finding. Examination with caliper reveals that rhythm is irregular.

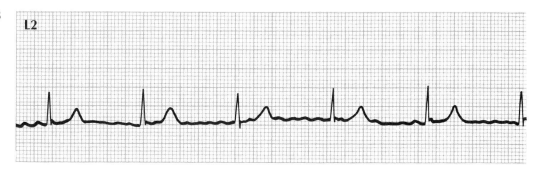

L2

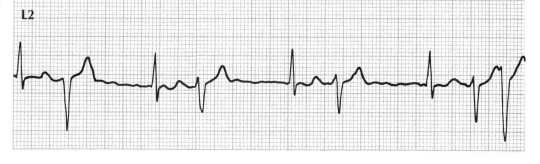

L2

38 Atrial Fibrillation with Junctional Rhythm:

Although the rhythm is regular, it should not be mistaken for sinus rhythm. The f wave is easily seen. The fifth QRS is preceded by the f wave which superficially resembles the P wave. The ventricular rate is 58. The QRS is narrow, therefore it is of junctional origin.

39 Atrial Fibrillation with Junctional Escape Rhythm and Premature Ventricular Complexes:

The basic rhythm is atrial fibrillation where f waves are well seen. Complexes 2, 4, 6, 8, and 9 are PVCs and the remaining beats are junctional.

40

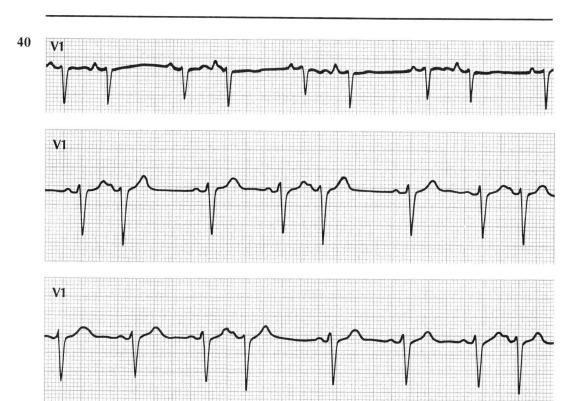

40 Atrial Premature Complexes with Bigeminy, Trigeminy, and Quadrigeminy:

PACs are noted every other beat (bigeminy) in the upper strip, every third beat (trigeminy) in the middle strip, and every fourth beat (quadrigeminy) in the lower strip.

41

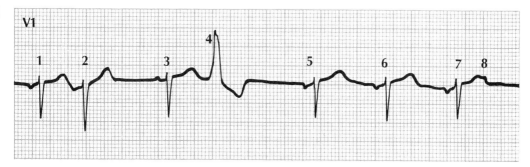

42

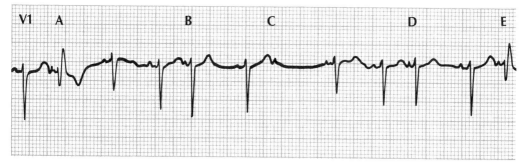

41 Atrial Escape and Blocked Premature Atrial Complex:

Complex 3 is an atrial escape. The P wave differs from the first, fifth, sixth, and seventh P wave which represent the basic sinus rhythm. There is blocked PAC (8) deforming the last T wave. A conducted PAC (2) and PVC (4) are also noted.

42 Premature Atrial Complexes With and Without Aberrancy:

A and E show aberrant conduction. B and D show normal conduction. C denotes blocked PAC.

43

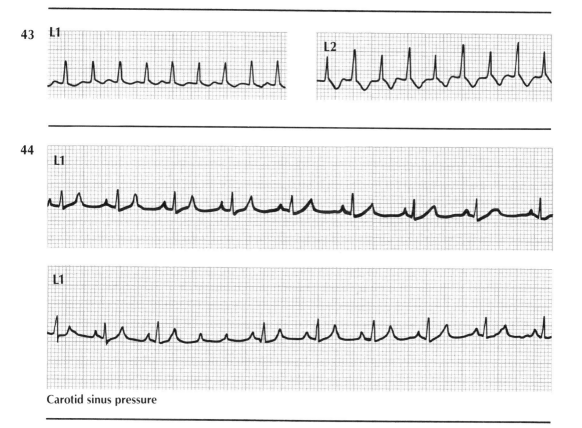

44

Carotid sinus pressure

43 Supraventricular Tachycardia With Electrical Alternans:

Lead 2 shows the electrical alternans where every other QRS is smaller than the preceding QRS complex. The most common cause of electrical alternans is malignant pericardial effusion.

44 Atrial Tachycardia with 2:1 AV Block:

The atrial rate is 200. The ventricular rate is 100.*

*Carotid sinus pressure uncovers the P wave which is lost in the T wave.

45

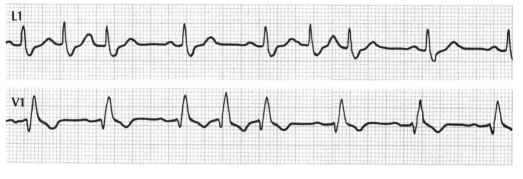

L1

V1

46

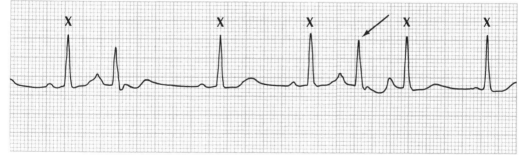

X X X X X

45 Interpolated Premature Junctional Complexes:

The second and the sixth complexes in the upper strip and the fourth complex in the lower strip are interpolated premature junctional contractions because each is sandwiched between two basic beats without disturbing the basic rhythm. There is also RBBB. Concealed conduction prolongs the PR interval after each interpolated complex. Note difference in the T wave of the interpolated complex when compared to normal complex.

46 Interpolated Premature Atrial Complex:

The arrow (←) indicates a sandwiched beat between two regular sinus beats, and is preceded by a P wave without disturbing the basic rhythm (X). The second beat is a PAC followed by a noncompensatory pause.

47

L2

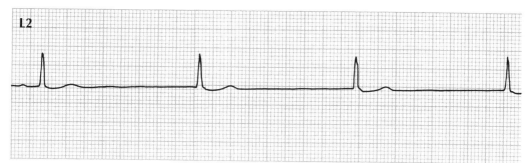

48

L2

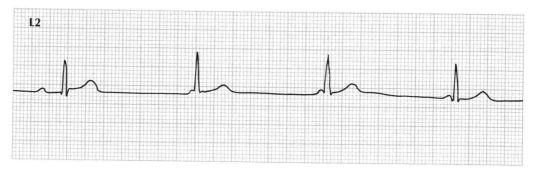

47 Junctional Escape Rhythm:

The first complex is sinus and the last three are junctional escape complexes where the QRS complexes are narrow and not preceded by P waves. The rate is 36.

48 Sinus Bradycardia With Junctional Escape:

The first P wave is conducted with first degree AV block (PR .26). Junctional escape follows, as the inherent junctional rate is slightly faster than the SA node. The last three P waves are not conducted even though they occur just prior to QRS complexes. This is also called incomplete AV dissociation.

49

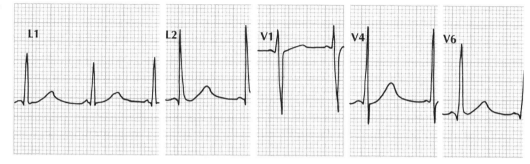

50

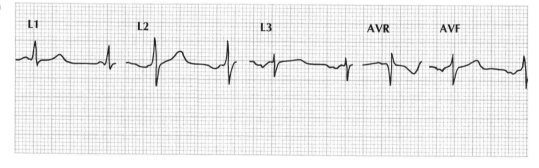

49 Coronary Nodal Rhythm:

Every QRS is preceded by P wave. The PR interval is less than .12 second. If the rhythm were associated with paroxysmal tachycardia, it would be called the LGL syndrome (Lown-Ganong-Levine).

50 Coronary Sinus Rhythm:

The P waves are inverted in leads 2, 3, and AVF, and upright in leads 1 and AVR. The duration of the PR interval is longer than .12 second. If the PR interval were .12 second or less, the rhythm would be called junctional (high nodal). If the P wave were inverted in lead 1, the rhythm would be called left atrial rhythm.

SECTION III

VENTRICULAR ARRHYTHMIAS

51

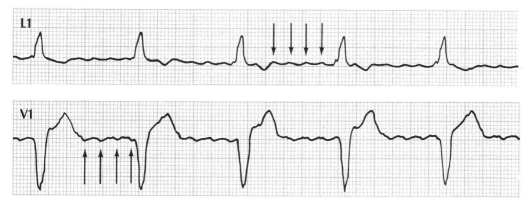

52

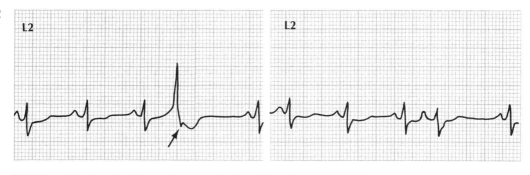

51 Atrial Flutter With Complete Heart Block and Accelerated Idioventricular Rhythm:

The atrial rate is 333.* The ventricular rate is 54 and the rhythm is regular. The QRS complexes are wide and there is no consistent relationship between F wave (↓↑) and QRS complexes.

*which puts it in flutter range than atrial fibrillation.

52 Premature Ventricular Complex:

The fourth QRS in the first strip is a PVC. The notch following the R wave (arrow) is a retrograde P wave. Note that the postectopic pause is noncompensatory. It is common for a PVC with a retrograde P wave not to have a compensatory pause because atrial depolarization resets the sinus node. The fourth beat in the second strip (from the same patient) is a PAC.

53

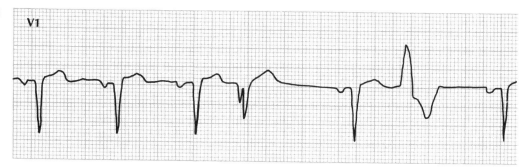

54

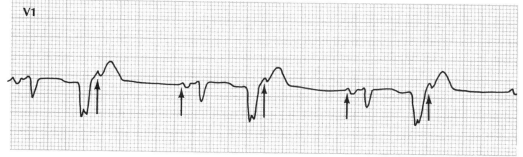

53 Multiform Premature Ventricular Complex:

The fourth QRS is a PVC with LBBB configuration and originates in the right ventricle. The sixth QRS is a PVC with RBBB configuration and originates in the left ventricle.

54 Ventricular Bigeminy:

The atrial rate (arrows) is 65. The PVCs do not disturb the P wave sequence. The P wave falling on the T wave of the PVC is blocked, as the AV node is refractory at that point. A retrograde P wave from the PVC almost always disturbs the P sequence (see strip 52).

55

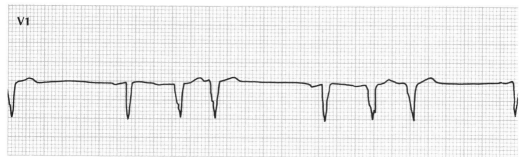

56

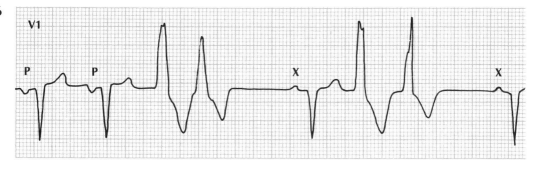

55 Ventricular Trigeminy:

The first complex of the trigeminy is sinus, followed by two paired PVCs. More often trigeminy consists of two sinus complexes and one PVC.

56 Premature Ventricular Complexes With Pairing:

Compare the ectopic P waves (X) after the PVCs with the normal P waves (P).

57

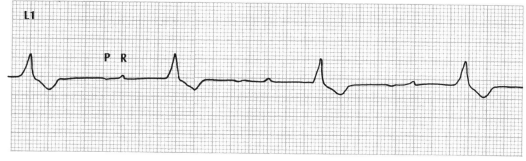

L1

P R

58

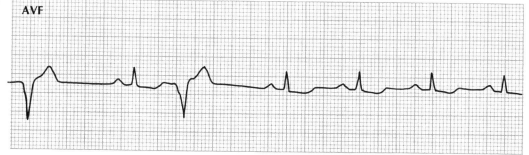

AVF

Strips 57 and 58 are from the same patient.

57 Ventricular Bigeminy:

The normal QRS complexes appear quite small using this lead. The first P wave, labeled P, is followed by a QRS labeled R. The more obvious QRS complexes are PVCs. This rhythm could be confused with first degree AV block if the QRS complex (R) is mistaken for a P wave.

58 Premature Ventricular Complexes:

Same patient as strip 57. The normal QRS complexes are more apparent in lead AVF than in lead 1.

59

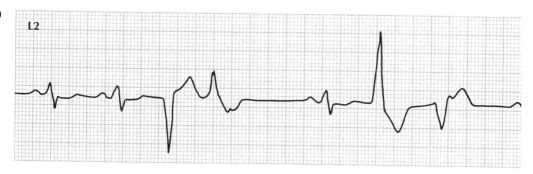

60

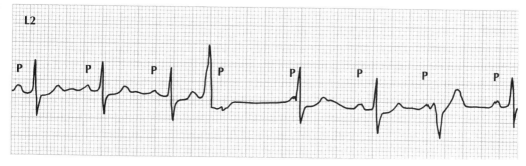

59 Multiform Premature Ventricular Complexes:

The third, fourth, sixth, and seventh QRS complexes are multiform PVCs. They are dissimilar in configuration, and the coupling intervals are variable. PVCs originating in the same ventricular focus may have different configurations, so the term multiform is preferred over multifocal.

60 End-Diastolic Premature Ventricular Complex:

The seventh QRS complex is an end-diastolic PVC, as it occurs after the onset of the sinus P wave. If differs from a PAC with aberrancy because the P wave (P) is not premature. The end-diastolic PVC is the least malignant of all forms of PVCs. The fourth QRS complex is a mid-diastolic PVC, and the fifth is a premature junctional beat. Neither disturbs atrial depolarization, as the PP interval is not altered.

61

L2

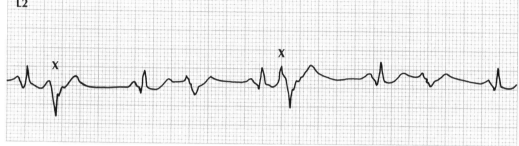

62

V1

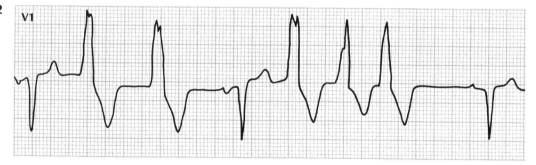

61 R on T Phenomenon:

This strip shows four PVCs. The second and sixth QRSs (X) are malignant PVCs, as they fall on the T wave (vulnerable zone) of the previous beat (R on T phenomenon). These PVCs may initiate ventricular tachycardia or ventricular fibrillation.

62 Ventricular Group Complexes (two and three consecutive PVCs):

The second group would be considered a short run of ventricular tachycardia since it contains three or more consecutive PVCs. The last P wave has a different configuration from the other P waves and probably represents atrial escape after the run of VT.

63

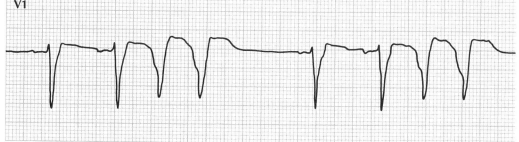

64

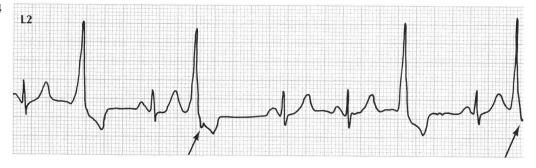

63 Ventricular Quadrigeminy:

This is a rare PVC sequence. A pair of PVCs follows a pair of sinus complexes repeatedly.

64 Premature Ventricular Complexes With Different Coupling Intervals:

The second and seventh QRS complexes have longer coupling intervals than the fourth and ninth complexes. A parasystolic focus should be ruled out. P waves (arrows) are noted in the T waves of the fourth and ninth complexes and indicate either blocked antegrade conduction or retrograde conduction.

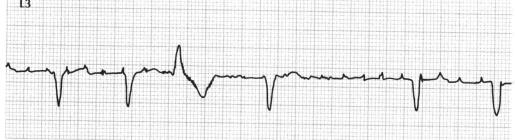

65

L3

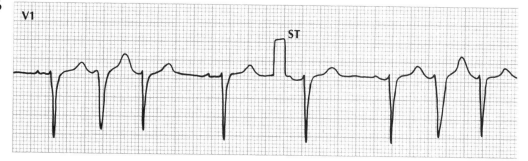

66

V1

ST

65 Premature Ventricular Complex With Atrial Fibrillation:

The rhythm is atrial fibrillation but the artifacts of muscle tremor make it resemble atrial flutter. The third QRS complex is a PVC, as it does not meet the criteria for Ashman phenomenon. If the third QRS is aberrant, then the last QRS complex should be aberrant because the ratio of the last RR cycle to the preceding one (22/40) is less than the ratio of the second RR cycle to the first one (13/19). Each small box counts as one when determining this ratio.

66 Interpolated Premature Ventricular Complexes:

The second and seventh QRS complexes are interpolated PVCs. These beats are true extrasystoles, as there is no compensatory pause and the cardiac rate is increased by their presence.

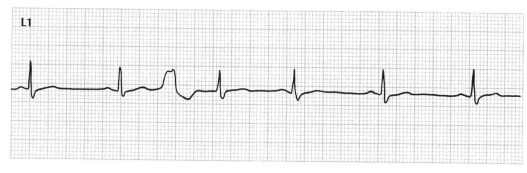

L1

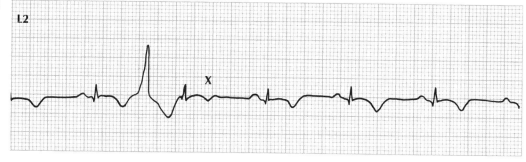

L2

X

67 Interpolated Premature Ventricular Complex with Concealed Conduction:

The third QRS complex is a PVC. There is no compensatory pause, but the PVC delays the onset of the following beat because of concealed conduction. The P wave of the P-QRS complex following the PVC is not clearly seen because it falls on the T wave of the PVC. The PR interval has increased because of concealed retrograde conduction that has made the AV node partially refractory.

68 Post-Premature Ventricular Complex T Wave Changes:

The third QRS complex is a PVC, and it is interpolated between two sinus complexes. The P wave of the fourth complex is buried in the preceding T wave. Note that the configuration of the T wave (X) of the fourth complex is dissimilar to the other T waves and represents altered repolarization.

69

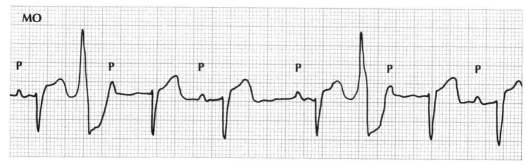

70

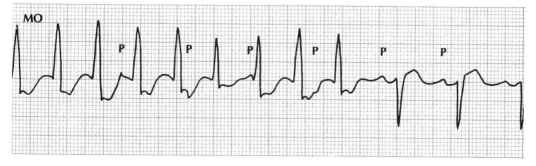

69 Interpolated Premature Ventricular Complexes With Concealed Conduction:

The second and sixth QRS complexes are PVCs, but they are interpolated as there is no compensatory pause. They each delay the following beat by concealed conduction. This patient has first degree AV block (PR .23), but after the PVC the concealed retrograde conduction of the AV node causes a further increase in the PR interval to .42. The P waves are marked (P).

70 Ventricular Tachycardia With Spontaneous Conversion to Sinus Rhythm:

Note that the ventricular rate of 140 does not interfere with the atrial rate of 85 during the episode of ventricular tachycardia. The QRS measures .12 second and has a different configuration from the normal sinus beat. The P waves are marked (P).

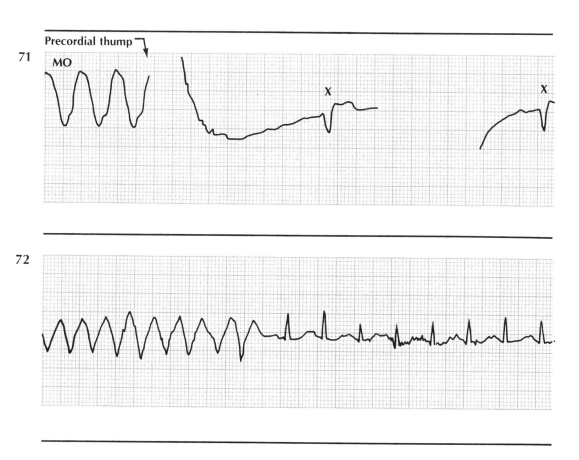

Precordial thump

71 MO

x

x

72

71 Ventricular Tachycardia With Conversion by Precordial Thump:

The ventricular rate during the VT is 160. Two sinus escape complexes (X) are noted following conversion.

72 Exercise-Induced Ventricular Tachycardia:

This arrhythmia was recorded during an exercise test. The VT had a rate of 250 and converted to sinus by cessation of the exercise. This is a serious abnormality, and the patient should be placed on anti-arrhythmic drugs.

73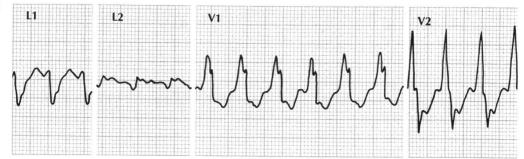

74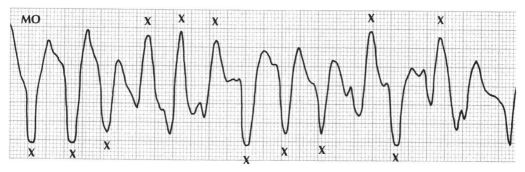

73 Supraventricular Versus Ventricular Tachycardia:

This is a difficult case. Carotid massage was tried without effect. The rhythm was converted to sinus by DC shock. This rhythm is most likely VT but supraventricular tachycardia with RBBB cannot be ruled out.

74 Bidirectional Ventricular Tachycardia:

The upper Xs denote VT with rate of 160, whereas the lower Xs denote VT with rate of 140.

75

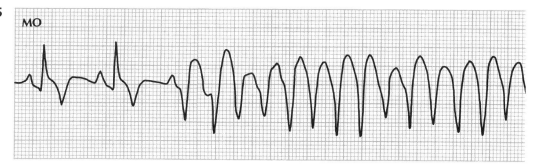

MO

76

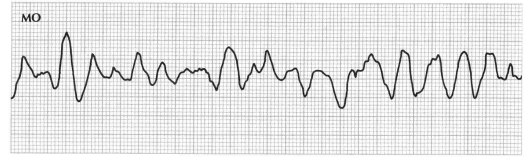

MO

75 Ventricular Tachycardia:

The VT with heart rate 230 started with an end-diastolic PVC.

76 Ventricular Fibrillation:

There is complete distortion and irregularity of all complexes.

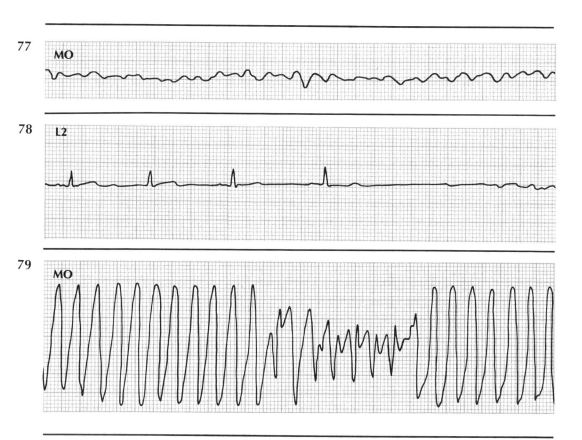

77 MO

78 L2

79 MO

77 Ventricular Fibrillation:

The complexes have smaller amplitude than in strip 85. A similar tracing could be obtained with loose monitor leads in a normal patient. However, no pulse would be noted in the patient with VF.

78 Cardiac Arrest:

The strip shows sinus arrest followed by ventricular standstill and then ventricular fibrillation.

79 Ventricular Flutter:

The ventricular rate is 300. Ventricular tachycardia rarely has a rate over 250. The ST segment and T wave cannot be recognized. Looking at the tracing upside down does not make much difference. The QRS complexes are tall, and the rhythm is regular. The seven QRS complexes in the middle of the strip also should be regarded as ventricular flutter because the rate is 300.

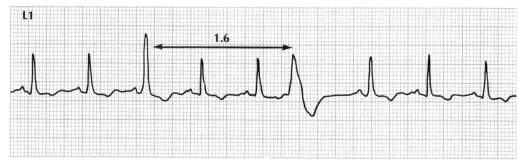

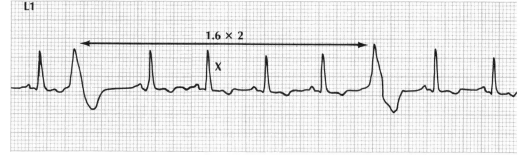

Strips 80 and 81 overlap.

80 Ventricular Parasystole:

The third and sixth QRS complexes originate from a parasystolic focus. The third is a fusion beat, as the ventricular parasystole and the normally conducted beat occur at the same time. Fusion complexes confirm the fact that there are two separate foci initiating ventricular depolarization.

81 Ventricular Parasystole:

Strips 80 and 81 overlap. The last five complexes of strip 80 are the same as the initial five complexes of strip 81. Long rhythm strips are needed to confirm the diagnosis of parasystole. The parasystolic focus discharges at a rate of 37.5, as the common denominator of the parasystolic focus is 1.6 second. The parasystolic focus is blocked if it occurs during the absolute refractory period (X). The variation in coupling intervals should make the reader suspicious of parasystole.

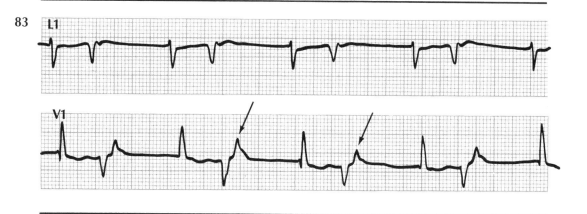

82 L2

83 L1

V1

82 Interpolated Premature Ventricular Complex Without Concealed Conduction:

An interpolated PVC is usually associated with concealed conduction.* This case is an exception where the P wave following the interpolated PVC is not disturbed. The second PVC is not interpolated.

*and the PR interval is longer in the complex after the PVC when compared to the complex before the interpolated PVC.

83 Ventricular Bigeminy With Concealed Conduction:

Every other complex is a premature ventricular complex. There is a P wave in the top of the T wave of each PVC (↓) with a significant delay of the conduction between the P wave and the QRS complex following it (0.72 sec). Delaying the conduction between P and QRS by a preceding QRS is called concealed conduction and is caused by partial retrograde depolarization of the AV node. This strip could be mistakened for junctional rhythm, when it is actually sinus with first degree block.

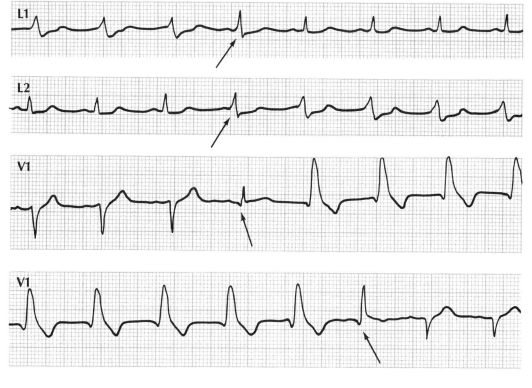

84 Fusion Complexes:

These strips show beautifully the disappearance and appearance of the accelerated idioventricular rhythm as it alternates with sinus rhythm. The arrows indicate fusion beats at the time of conversion from one rhythm to another. The fusion complex combines the features of the normal QRS with idioventricular QRS.

Intravenous lidocaine

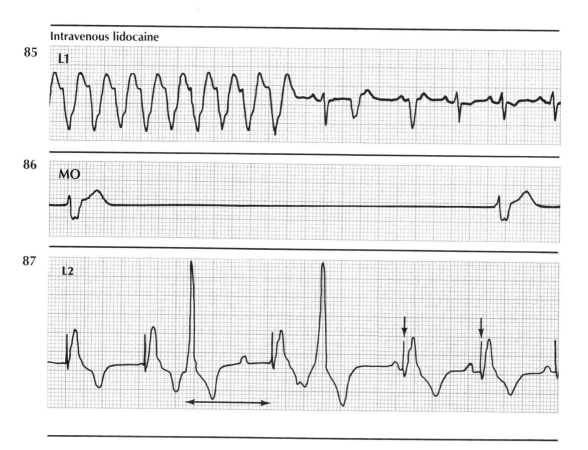

85 L1

86 MO

87 L2

85 Ventricular Tachycardia:

Injection of intravenous lidocaine converted this arrhythmia to sinus rhythm, making the diagnosis of VT most likely because lidocaine does not usually convert supraventricular tachycardia with aberrancy to sinus rhythm.

86 Idioventricular Rhythm:

The wide QRS complexes represent ventricular escape. The heart rate is 13 (4.7 seconds between complexes). This patient required an artificial pacemaker.

87 Functioning Demand Pacemaker:

The pacemaker is preset to fire at 70. The pacemaker is inhibited when it senses the third beat, a premature ventricular complex. The interval between the sensed complex and the next pacemaker spike is called the escape interval (lower, horizontal arrow), which is usually slightly longer (.92 second) then the automated interval (.84 second). The automated interval is the period between two consecutive pacemaker-driven complexes (upper arrows).

88

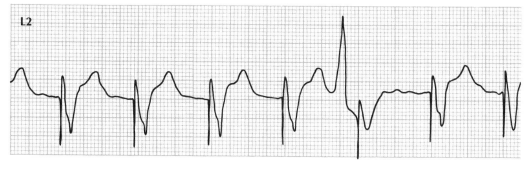

89

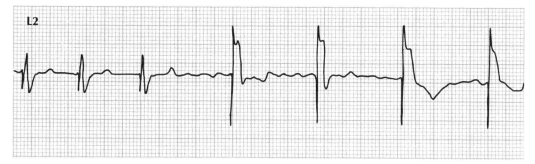

88 Fixed Rate Pacemaker:

Note that the fifth pacemaker spike falls on the T wave of the PVC. In this case, this is not a pacemaker malfunction. However, if this were a demand pacemaker this phenomenon would represent malfunction of the sensing mechanism.

89 R-Triggered Demand Pacemaker:

The basic rhythm is atrial fibrillation as evidenced by the f waves and irregularity of the RR intervals. The first three QRS complexes are spontaneous and trigger the pacemaker spike. The last four QRS complexes are pacemaker-induced at a rate of 65. The period between the third and fourth spike is the escape interval.

90

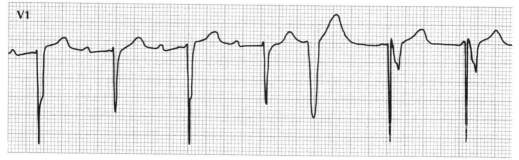

91

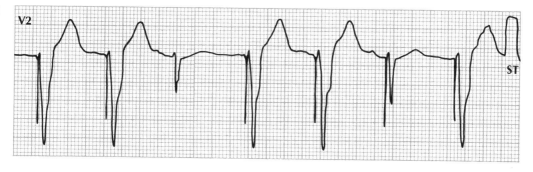

90 Functioning Demand Pacemaker:

The pacemaker is preset to fire at 70. The second and fourth complexes are normal sinus complexes. The first and third complexes are also sinus but the pacemaker fires on the R wave. As the pacemaker rate and the spontaneous rate are very similar, the compensatory pause after the PVC (fifth complex) activates the demand pacemaker. First degree AV block is also present (PR .28).

91 Functioning Demand Pacemaker:

The third complex is a sinus complex, and the sixth is a fusion complex. The remainder of the complexes are pacemaker-induced.

92

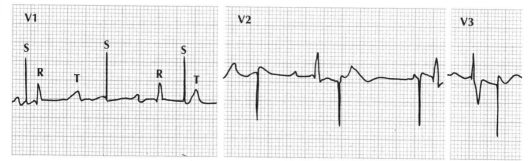

93

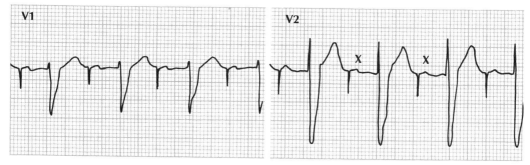

92 Malfunctioning Demand Pacemaker:

The demand pacemaker is firing at a rate of 70, but does not capture the ventricle. It continues to fire at 70 regardless of the spontaneous beats. This indicates that the sensing function is also impaired. (S denotes pacemaker spike, R denotes QRS complex, and T denotes T wave.)

93 Atrial Pacemaker:

Since the tip of the pacemaker is located in the atrium, every pacemaker spike is followed by a P wave (X).

94

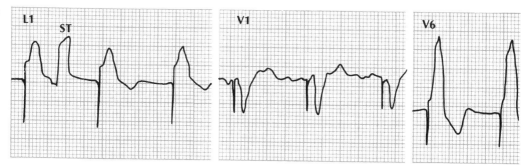

95

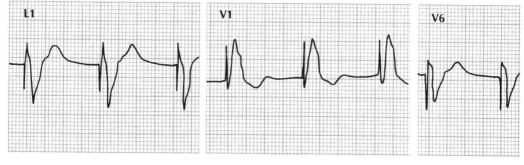

94 Unipolar Right Ventricular Pacemaker:

One electrode is in the right ventricle and the other is at a remote spot in the chest. The current travels a relatively long distance from one electrode to the other; hence the pacemaker spike is relatively tall. When the pacemaker tip is in the right ventricular apex, the QRS complex resembles LBBB, as the left ventricle is depolarized after the right ventricle.

95 Unipolar Left Ventricular Pacemaker:

The QRS complexes have the configuration of RBBB, as the right ventricle is depolarized after the left ventricle.

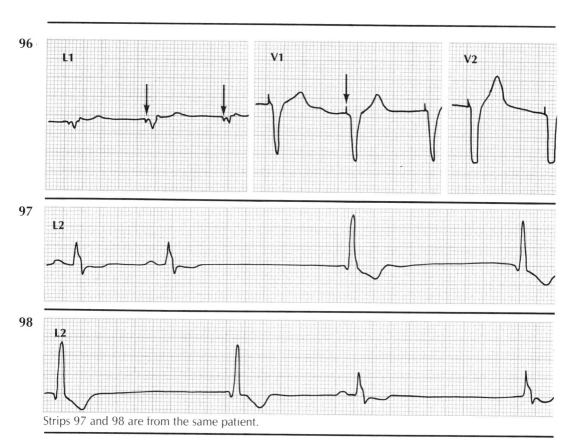

Strips 97 and 98 are from the same patient.

96 Bipolar Right Ventricular Pacemaker:

When both electrodes are located in the right ventricle the current does not have to travel as far, so the pacemaker spike (arrows) is relatively short.

97 Ventricular Escape Complexes:

The first two QRS complexes are of sinus origin. The last two QRS complexes are of ventricular origin with rate of 33. The features of ventricular escape complex are: (A) no P wave preceding QRS, (B) QRS duration of .12 second or longer, (C) bizarre QRS configuration, and (D) slow rate. In this example the QRS duration of the sinus complex is .12 second because of an associated bundle branch block.

98 Ventricular and Junctional Escape Complexes:

Same patient as strip 97, but the strips are not continuous. The first and second QRS complexes are ventricular escape complexes. The third complex is of sinus origin. The last complex is a junctional escape complex. If the number of consecutive ventricular complexes were three or more they would be called idioventricular rhythm.

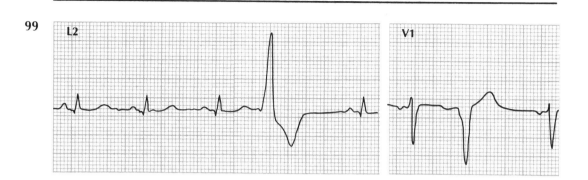

99 L2   V1

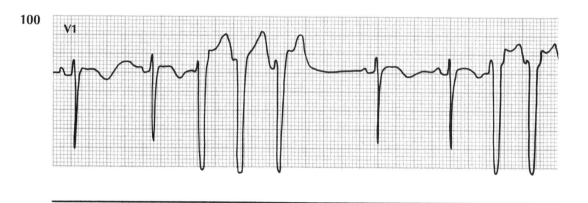

100 V1

99 Premature Ventricular Complexes:

The fourth complex in lead 2 and the second complex in V1 are PVCs.

100 Paroxysmal Ventricular Tachycardia Due to Prolongation of QT Interval:

This combination can be seen in rare congenital syndromes, quinidine excess, and hypokalemia. Note that the QT interval of the first complex is .56 second, and of the sixth complex is .48 second. (The upper limit for QT interval in heart rate of 70 is .41 second.)

101

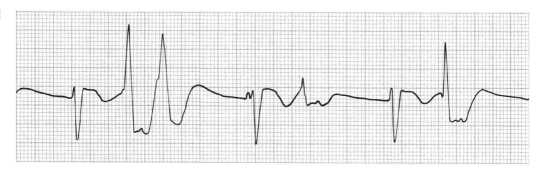

102

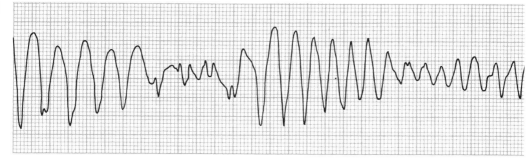

101 Multiform Premature Ventricular Complexes:

The background rhythm is junctional with marked prolongation of the QT interval to 680 msec., secondary to procainamide and quinidine therapy. Note the retrograde P waves in the depressed ST segments of the PVC's. This patient later developed torsades de pointes.

102 Torsades de Pointes:

A form of ventricular tachycardia characterized by wide QRS complexes of changing amplitude that appear to twist around the isoelectric baseline. The term, torsades de pointes, (twistings of the points) connotes a syndrome, as it occurs in the setting of prolonged ventricular repolarization with QT intervals exceeding 500 msec.

SECTION IV

DISORDERS
OF
CONDUCTION

103

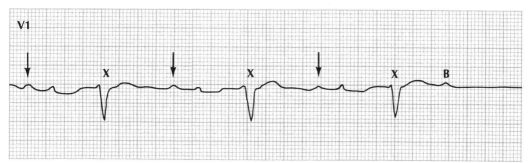

103 First Degree AV Block:

The PR interval is .30 second. Ventricular bigeminy is present as every other QRS complex is a PVC (denoted by X). The arrows denote P waves followed by QRS complexes of extremely low voltage. A different monitoring lead might help to clarify the interpretation. B denotes a blocked PAC where the P wave is premature and not followed by a QRS.

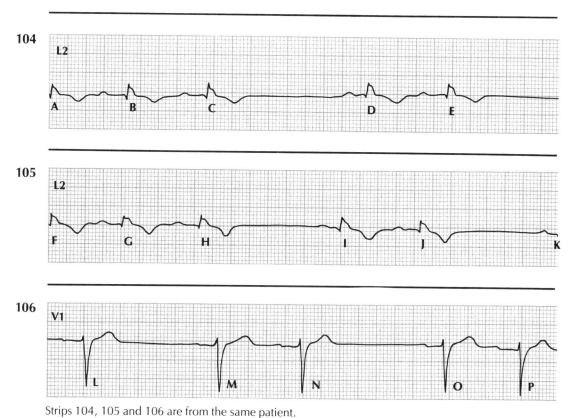

104   L2

A   B   C   D   E

105   L2

F   G   H   I   J   K

106   V1

L   M   N   O   P

Strips 104, 105 and 106 are from the same patient.

104 Sinus Block:

The basic rhythm is sinus with heart rate of 70 (AB, BC, and DE). However, CD is twice as long as BC or DE. The P wave is not seen following complex C and complex E. Note also that the first degree AV block (PR .30) improves after the long pause (PR .23) before D, indicating partial recovery of the AV node. This patient most likely has sick sinus syndrome (SSS).

105 Sinus Block:

Same patient as strip 104, but the strips are not continuous. The HI and JK intervals are less than twice the previous PP intervals. Small changes in the PP interval may be accounted for by respiratory sinus arrhythmia. First degree AV block (PR .24) becomes normal (PR .19) after the long pause.

106 Sinus Arrest:

Same patient as strips 104 and 105. This strip could be confused with sinus bradycardia with atrial bigeminy (N and P). However, the long pauses (LM and NO) are not a multiple of the normal heartbeat cycle length (MN and OP), and the variation is too great to be accounted for by sinus arrhythmia.

107

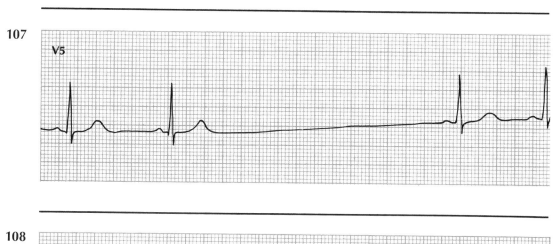

108

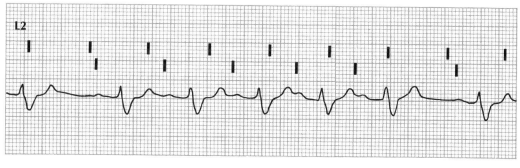

107 Sinus Arrest:

The long pause (3.2 seconds) has no relationship to the PP interval of the basic rhythm. It is less than three times the previous PP cycle and more than three times the succeeding PP cycle. However, it may be argued that in the presence of sinus arrhythmia this long pause may be sinus block, because the long pause is three times the average basic PP cycle. In either case, the patient has sick sinus syndrome and should be treated with a pacemaker.

108 Second Degree Sinus Block, Type I (Wenckebach):

There is gradual shortening of PP intervals followed by a long PP interval not exceeding two times the previous one. The upper verticle lines denote the assumed onset of the sinus impulse, and the lower verticle lines denote the onset of the atrial impulse. Note the gradual prolongation of the SP interval (from sinus impulse to the beginning of the P wave) until the sinus impulse is blocked completely (6:5 block). In this particular example, the last PP interval before the pause does not show significant change. This rhythm terminology should not be confused with second degree AV block, Mobitz Type I (Wenckebach), where the PR interval gradually lengthens until a beat is blocked completely. In this tracing the PR interval does not change.

109

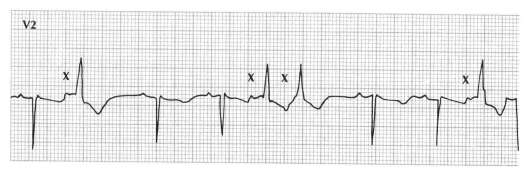

V2

During carotid massage

110

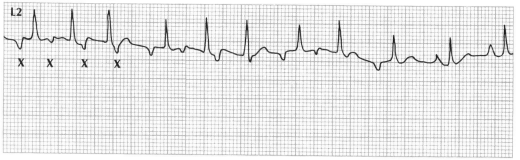

L2

109 Premature Atrial Complexes With Aberrancy:

The second, fifth, sixth, and ninth complexes show aberrant conduction. They are conducted via the left bundle branch giving the configuration of right bundle branch block in lead V2. Each is preceded by a premature P wave (marked X). These aberrant beats could be confused with premature ventricular contractions if the preceding P waves are not noticed.

110 Atrial Tachycardia With Wenckebach AV Block:

The first PR interval of each Wenckebach cycle is longer than .12 second. Note the progressive prolongation of the PR interval until a blocked P wave occurs. The Xs mark the inverted P waves of the first Wenckebach cycle. The RR intervals become progressively shorter in the Wenckebach cycle. The rhythm converts to sinus (last two complexes by carotid massage. Because the P waves are inverted in lead 2, this rhythm may be classified as coronary sinus tachycardia.

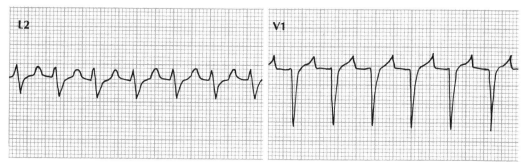

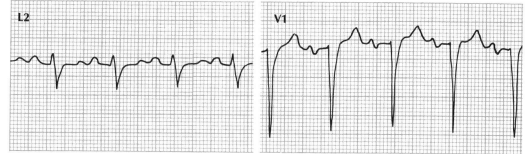

Strips 111 and 112 are from the same patient.

111 Sinus Tachycardia With First Degree AV Block:

The atrial rate is 140. The P waves are superimposed on the preceding T waves and are more apparent in lead V1. The PR interval of .24 second indicates first degree AV block. Since normal T waves are not available for comparison, a diagnosis of junctional tachycardia could be entertained.

112 First Degree AV Block:

Same patient as strip 111. The PR interval is prolonged to .24 second. The T waves (L2 and V1) have a different configuration from those in strip 111, confirming the previous diagnosis of sinus tachycardia.

113

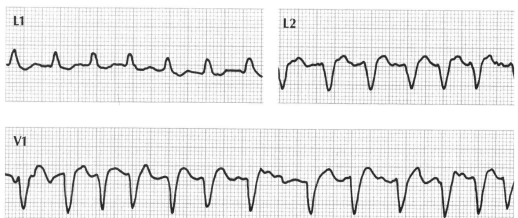

113 Atrial Fibrillation and Left Bundle Branch Block:

The rhythm is irregularly irregular with heart rate of 130. The QRS is wide. This strip should not be mistaken for ventricular tachycardia.

114

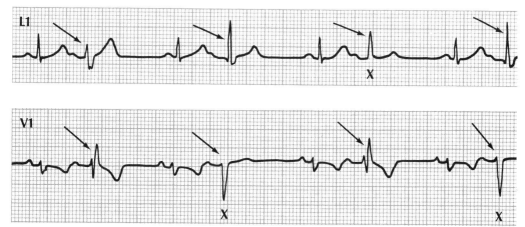

114 Premature Atrial Complexes With Variable Aberrancy:

There are at least three different forms of aberrancy here (→). RBBB is the most common type of aberrancy, but those complexes denoted by X do not have RBBB configuration.

115

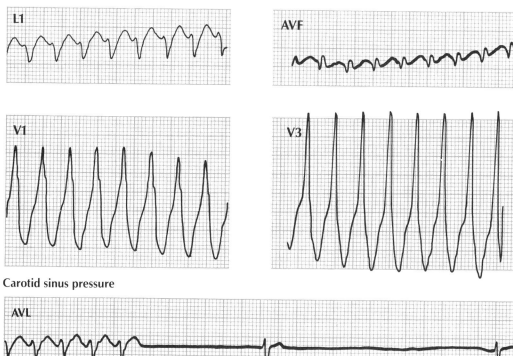

L1

AVF

V1

V3

Carotid sinus pressure

AVL

115 Supraventricular Tachycardia (SVT) With Aberrancy:

The rhythm may be mistaken for VT. In the lower strip, however, carotid massage was performed and caused marked slowing, making the diagnosis of SVT with aberrancy most likely because stimulation of the vagus nerve does not usually convert VT.

116

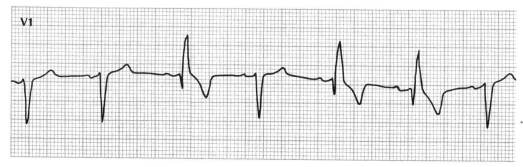

117

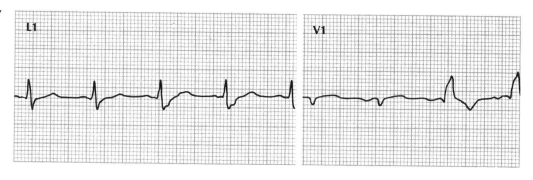

116 Aberrant Conduction:

The third, fifth, and sixth complexes have the configuration of RBBB and are each preceded by a P wave.

117 Intermittent Right Bundle Branch Block:

The last three complexes of lead 1 and the last two complexes of lead V1 have the configuration of RBBB without change of the heart rate. This should not be mistaken for an end-diastolic PVC where the QRS occurs after the P wave but the PR interval is shorter.

118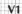

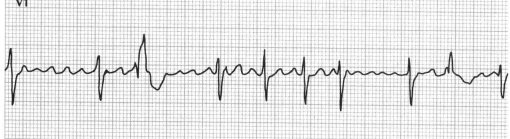

119

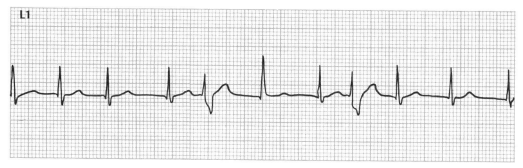

118 Ashman Phenomenon:

Aberrant conduction is difficult to diagnose in atrial fibrillation because P waves are absent. Aberration should be considered if the beat in question follows a short RR cycle that follows a long cycle. The ratio of short cycle to long should be less than any ratio of two consecutive RR cycles without aberrancy. In 80 percent of the cases, the configuration of the aberrant QRS resembles RBBB. There is usually a variable coupling interval with aberration, while with a PVC the coupling interval is usually constant. In this strip the third and ninth QRS complexes are aberrant.

119 Aberrant Conduction:

Atrial fibrillation is present. The fifth and eighth QRS complexes are aberrant. They follow the rule of Ashman phenomenon (see strip 118.)

120

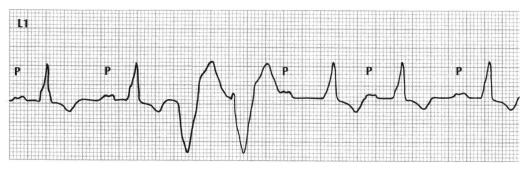

L1

P P P P P

121

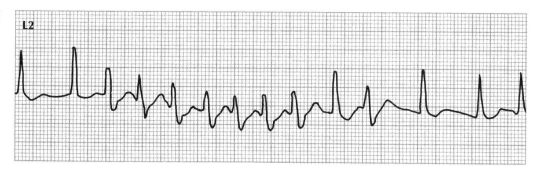

L2

120 Concealed Conduction:

The basic rhythm is sinus with rate of 62. First degree AV block is present. The third and fourth QRS complexes are consecutive PVCs followed by a P wave (P) that is conducted but with a longer PR interval (PR .44) than usual (PR .28). This pronounced delay of the PR interval is due to concealed retrograde conduction of the AV node from the preceding PVC.

121 Aberrant Conduction:

Atrial fibrillation is present, as the background rhythm is irregularly irregular. There is a run of seven aberrant QRS complexes of similar configuration. The first one follows a short RR interval after a long RR interval (Ashman phenomenon). The 11th QRS complex is aberrant too, as it is similar to the other aberrant QRS complexes in configuration.

122

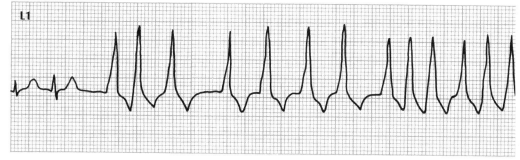

123

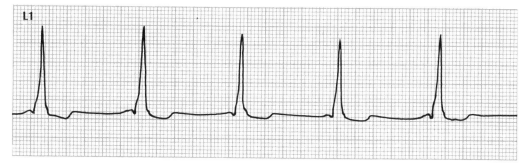

Strips 122 and 123 are from the same patient.

122 Wolff-Parkinson-White Syndrome:

The background rhythm is atrial fibrillation, as the rhythm is irregularly irregular. The first two QRS complexes are conducted normally. The remainder are conducted via the accessory bundle. The slurred upstroke of the QRS is the delta wave. The extremely rapid rate of the last six compleses (over 200) is unusual for supraventricular rhythm except in pre-excitation syndrome. Also note that the third complex started after a long RR cycle, which distinguishes it from Ashman phenomenon.

123 Wolff-Parkinson-White Syndrome:

This is a rhythm strip for the same patient (strip 122) when he has sinus rhythm. Note the short PR interval (.08), delta wave, and prolonged QRS (.14).

124

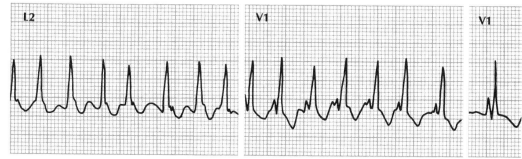

125

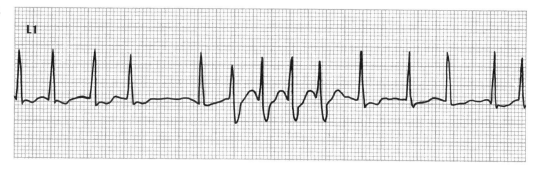

124 Right Bundle Branch Block:

The first and second strips show atrial fibrillation. The QRS complexes are wide and have the configuration of RBBB. The last strip shows a complex when the patient has sinus rhythm.

125 Aberrant Conduction:

Atrial fibrillation is present. The rhythm is irregularly irregular except the sixth, seventh, eighth, and ninth complexes, which are regular at heart rate 200 and suggest VT. But because the run meets the criteria for Ashman phenomenon (the preceding RR interval is short compared to the previous one), supraventricular tachycardia with aberrant conduction should be seriously considered.

126

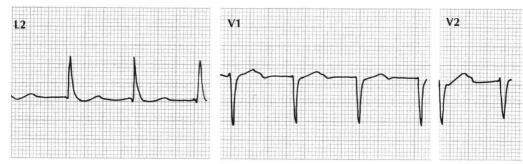

127

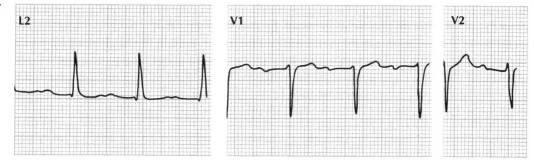

Strips 126 and 127 are from the same patient.

126 First Degree AV Block:

This strip superficially resembles junctional rhythm. P waves are superimposed on the T waves (PR .30), and are best seen in leads V1 and V2.

127 First Degree AV Block:

This strip was previously taken from the patient in strip 126. Here the first degree AV block is obvious, as there is a slight change in the ventricular rate and QT interval. In many cases, reviewing an old ECG is important to clarify an ambiguous arrhythmia.

During carotid massage

128

L2

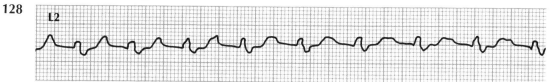

129

L2

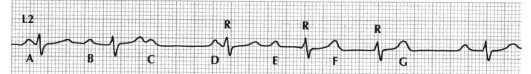

128 First Degree AV Block:

Effect of carotid massage on first degree AV block. The first three RR intervals may resemble junctional rhythm because the P wave is superimposed on the T wave. Carotid sinus pressure slowed the rate slightly and the P wave became apparent.

129 Wenckebach:

This patient also has second degree AV block, Mobitz Type I. The block changes from 3:2 (A, B, C) to 4:3 (D, E, F, G). Note the gradual shortening of the RR cycle (R, R, R), a characteristic feature of Wenckebach.

130

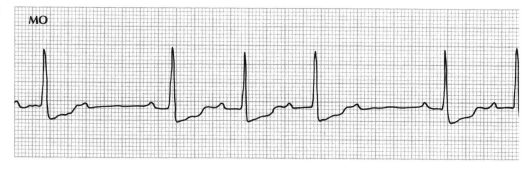

131

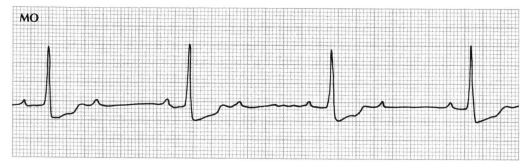

Strips 130 and 131 are from the same patient.

130 Wenckebach (second degree AV block, Mobitz Type I):
This patient has 4:3 block.

131 Wenckebach (second degree AV block, Mobitz Type I):
The block is 2:1. Same patient as strip 130, but the strips are not continuous. Without the previous strip, it would be impossible to tell whether this was Mobitz I or II.

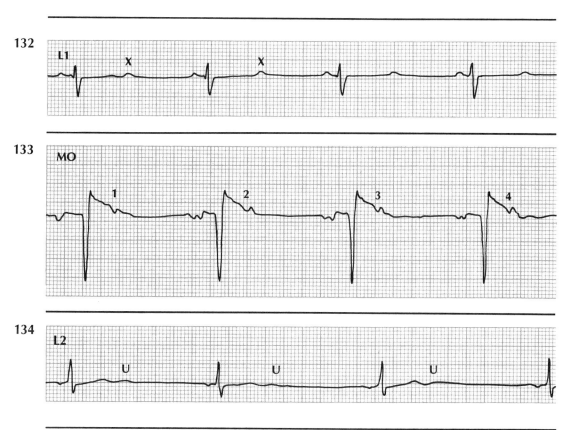

132 L1   X   X

133 MO   1   2   3   4

134 L2   U   U   U

132 Second Degree AV Block:

The atrial rate is 84, and the ventricular rate is 42. This tracing looks like Mobitz II, but the nonconducted P waves (X) could represent the dropped complexes of a short run of Wenckebach (Mobitz I). Bundle of His recordings would be useful to see if the block is above (Wenckebach) or below (Mobitz II) the bundle of His.

133 Blocked Premature Atrial Complexes:

This rhythm may superficially resemble second degree AV block. The prematurity of the blocked atrial contractions (1, 2, 3, 4) can be detected with calipers.

134 U Waves:

This patient has sinus bradycardia. The heart rate is 35. The U waves (U) may superficially resemble blocked P waves. Sinus arrhythmia is also present, so RR intervals and UU intervals are not equidistant.

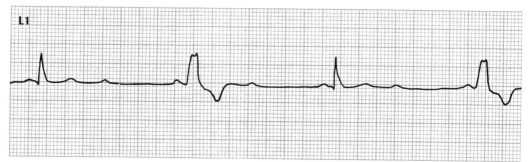

L1

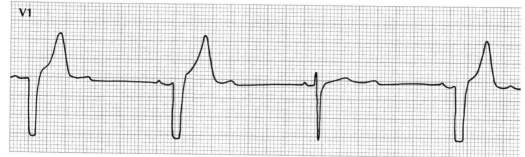

V1

Strips 135 and 136 are from the same patient.

135 Intermittent Left Bundle Branch Block:

Second degree AV block is present. The atrial rate is 75, and the ventricular rate is 37. The block is 2:1.

136 Intermittent Left Bundle Branch Block:

Same patient as strip 135. Second degree AV block (2:1) is present.

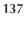

137

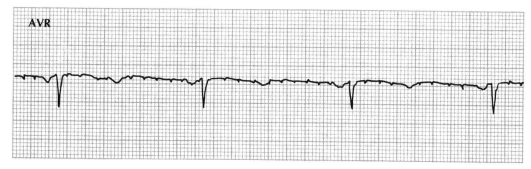

AVR

138

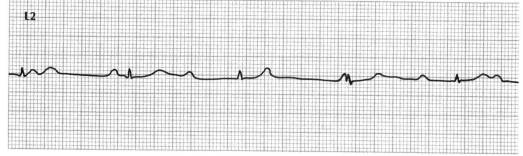

L2

137 Second Degree AV Block (2:1):

The atrial rate is 80, and the ventricular rate is 40. There is a muscle tremor artifact with rate of about 400.

138 Third Degree AV Block:

This is also called complete heart block. The atrial rate is 75, and the ventricular rate is 50. The QRS complexes are narrow (less than .10 second). Therefore, they are of junctional origin.

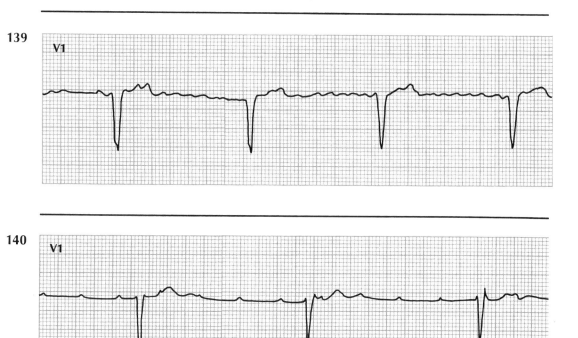

139   V1

140   V1

139 Atrial Fibrillation With Complete AV Block:

The ventricular rate is 43 and regular. The atrial rate is about 400. Digitalis toxicity should be suspected whenever AV dissociation is present.

140 Atrial Tachycardia With Complete AV Block:

The atrial rate is 140, and the ventricular rate is 33. None of the P waves is conducted.

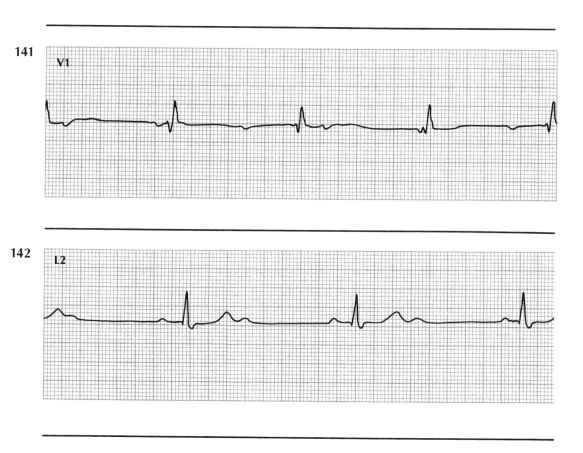

141 V1

142 L2

141 Third Degree AV Block With Ventriculophasic Sinus Arrhythmia:
The PP interval containing the QRS is shorter than the PP interval without the QRS. Compare the PP interval containing the third QRS complex with the PP interval following it.

142 Third Degree AV Block:
The atrial rate is 65, and the ventricular rate is 33. This rhythm strip could be confused with second degree AV block (2:1) if the gradual change of TP and PR intervals is not noticed. Ventriculophasic sinus arrhythmia is present.

143

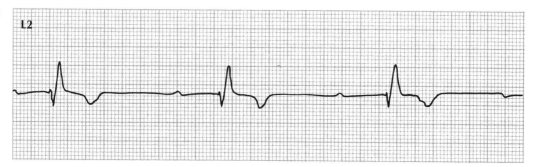

L2

144

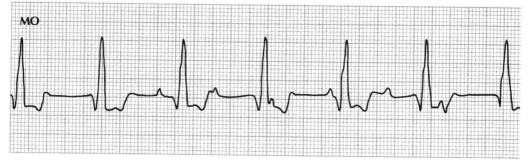

MO

143 Third Degree AV Block:

This could be confused with sinus bradycardia with first degree block if the superimposed P on T (third complex) and the changes in PR interval are not noticed.

144 Complete AV Block:

The atrial rate is 96, and the ventricular rate is 68. It is unusual for complete AV block to have a ventricular rate over 60, but this patient has been on isoproterenol. Note the gradual prolongation of the PR interval, causing a superficial resemblance to Wenckebach AV block, but there is no change in the RR interval.

145

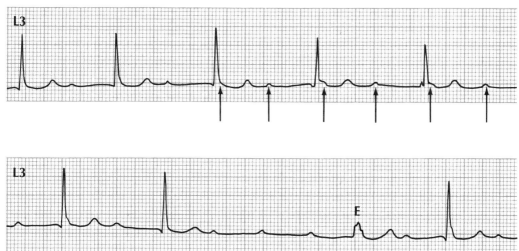

145 Sinus Tachycardia With AV Dissociation:

The atrial rate is 115. The ventricular rate is 53. The QRS complexes are of normal duration, suggesting junctional rhythm. There is no constant relation between the P wave and the QRS complex. There is a period of ventricular standstill. The third complex in the lower strip is a ventricular escape (E). This tracing was taken from a young man with a clinical diagnosis of myocarditis. A temporary pacemaker was inserted for three days and removed when the ECG returned to normal.

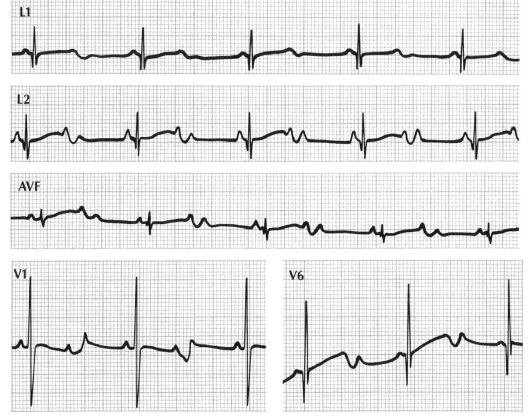

146 Blocked Premature Atrial Complexes:

This tracing is from a two year old boy with congenital bilateral cataracts and fainting spells. The PP intervals do not measure out. There is marked prolongation of the QT interval. The T wave could be mistaken for a P wave in some leads. The diagnosis of 2:1 AV block might be entertained if one did not use the caliper.

147

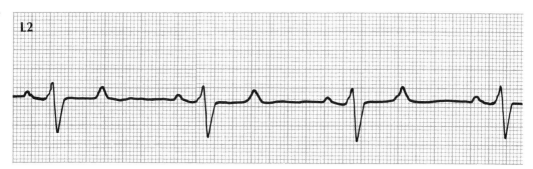

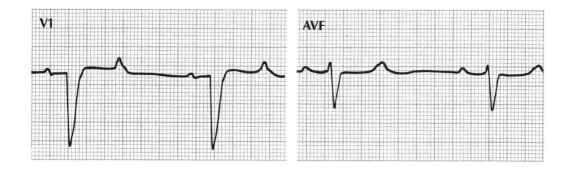

147 Second Degree AV Block:

The ventricular rate is 35 and the atrial rate is 70. This 2:1 block could be mistaken for sinus bradycardia because nonconducted P is buried in the T wave.

148

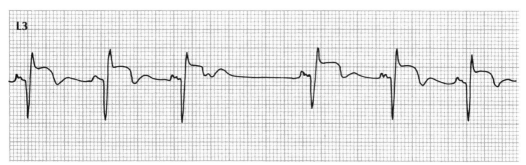

149

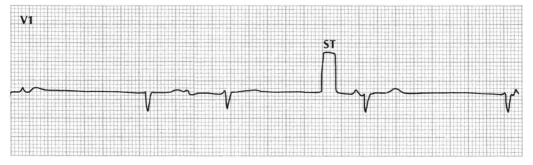

148 Blocked Premature Atrial Complex:

A P wave falls on the T wave of the third complex, and it is not followed by a QRS complex, since the AV node is still refractory.

149 Sinus Bradycardia With Incomplete AV Dissociation:

The atrial rate is 32, and the ventricular rate is 40. Only the second P wave is conducted (with the first degree AV block) making the AV dissociation incomplete. Slow antegrade conduction is possible, but retrograde block is complete.

150

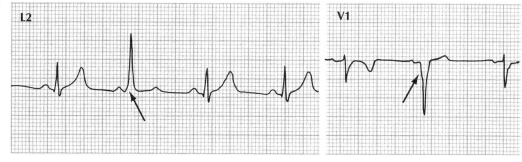

151

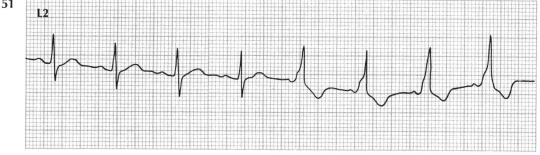

150 Intermittent Wolff-Parkinson-White Syndrome:
The second complex in leads 2 and V1 show delta waves, short PR intervals, and prolongation of the QRS.

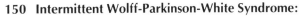

151 Wolff-Parkinson-White Syndrome:
The first four complexes are normally conducted. The last four compleses are conducted via the accessory bundle. Note the short PR interval, delta waves, and prolonged QRS.

152

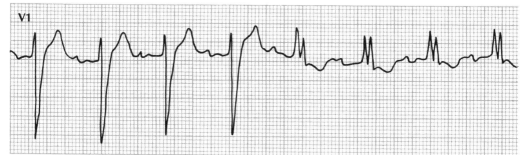

153

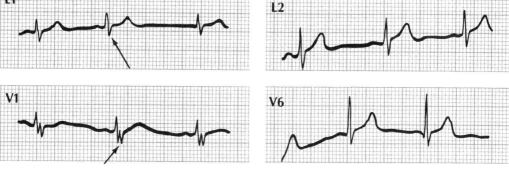

152 Alternating Bundle Branch Block:

The first four QRS complexes have the configuration of LBBB, whereas the last four QRS complexes have the configuration of RBBB. The strip also shows first degree AV block. This is an example of trifascicular block.

153 Incomplete Right Bundle Branch Block:

The QRS interval measures 0.10 sec in lead V1. Terminal slowing is noted in lead 1 (↑) and lead V1 (→). This tracing is from an asymptomatic eighteen year old man with normal cardiac auscultation and normal chest X-ray. IRBBB can be a normal variant electrocardiogram.

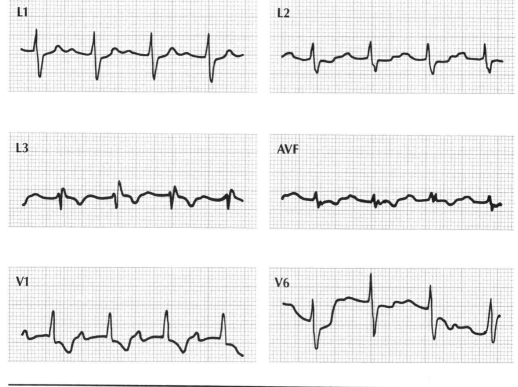

154

L1

L2

L3

AVF

V1

V6

154 Right Bundle Branch Block and First Degree AV Block:

The PR interval is markedly prolonged at 0.32 seconds. His bundle studies would be required to determine if this patient has monofascicular RBBB with block in AV node or trifascicular block with block below the AV node. The interval from atrial excitation to His spike (AH interval) is prolonged in the former, while the interval from the spike to ventricular excitation (HV interval) is prolonged in the latter.

155

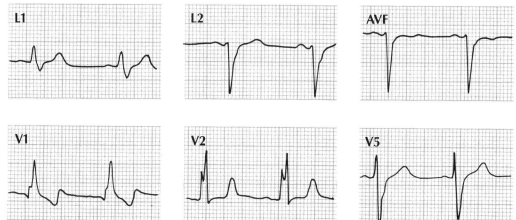

155 Right Bundle Branch Block and Left Anterior Hemiblock:

This patient has bifascicular block. With blockage of right bundle, and anterior division of left bundle, LAH should be suspected when QRS axis is more than -30°.

156

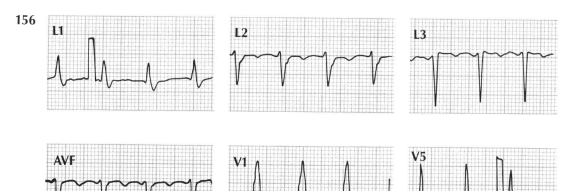

156 Right Bundle Branch Block, First Degree AV Block, and Left Anterior Hemiblock:
This patient has a high probability of having trifascicular block, which would be proved by His bundle studies if prolongation of HV interval is found (see strip 154).

157

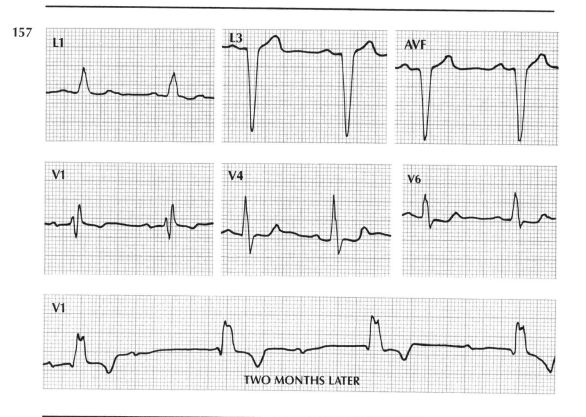

L1 L3 AVF

V1 V4 V6

V1

TWO MONTHS LATER

157 Right Bundle Branch Block, First Degree AV Block, and Left Anterior Hemiblock:
The diagnosis of trifascicular block was confirmed without His bundle studies when the patient developed complete heart block two months later (lower strip).

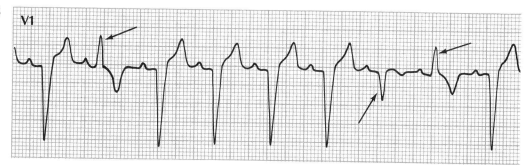

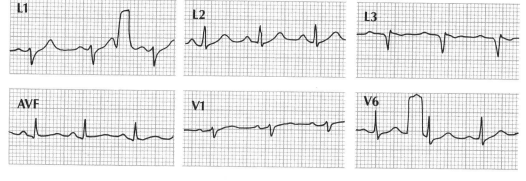

158 Bilateral Bundle Branch Block:

This patient has trifascicular block with intermittent LBBB and RBBB (←). Normal conduction (↑) is also noted.

159 Left Posterior Hemiblock:

When the QRS axis is more than +90° one should suspect blockage of the posterior division of the left bundle if RVH is not present. The ECG is from an asymptomatic 28 year old man.

160

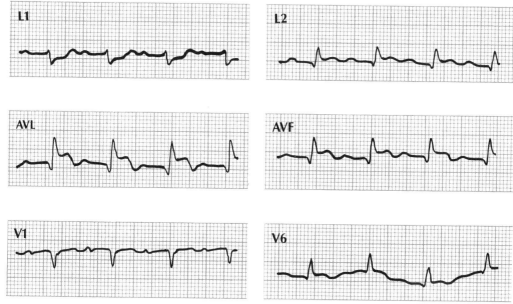

160 **Inferior Myocardial Infarction, Posterior Hemiblock, and First Degree AV Block:**
There is evidence of inferolateral myocardial infarction. The QRS axis is +140° and the PR interval is 0.03 second. His bundle studies would establish if trifascicular block (prolonged HV interval) or monofascicular block (normal HV interval) was present (see strip 154).

161

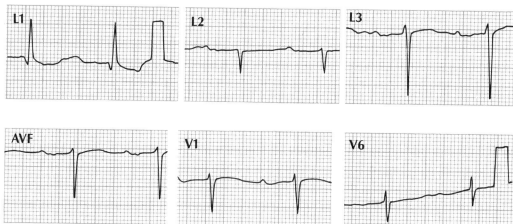

161 First Degree AV Block and Left Anterior Hemiblock:

The PR interval is 0.36 and the QRS axis is -45°. His bundle studies would establish diagnosis of trifascicular block (prolonged HV interval) or monofascicular block (prolonged AH interval) (see strip 154).

162

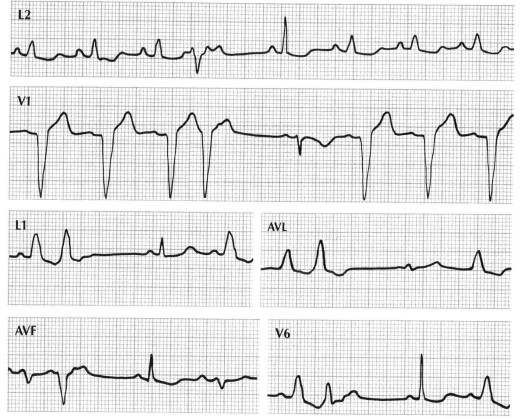

162 Intermittent Left Bundle Branch Block and Premature Ventricular Complexes:

The basic rhythm is sinus with LBBB. This rhythm is interrupted by premature ventricular complexes followed by normally conducted sinus beats. The postextrasystolic pause enables the left bundle to recover and conduct normally.

163

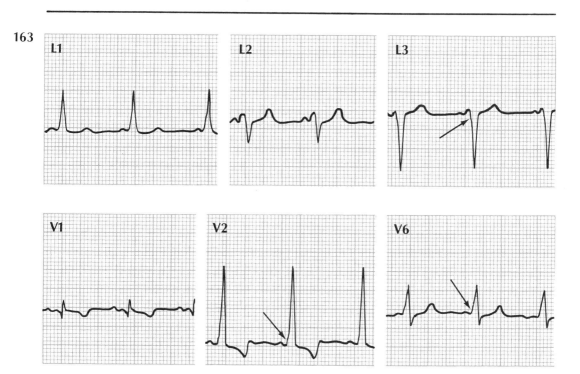

163 Wolff-Parkinson-White Syndrome:

PR interval is short. Delta wave is present (→) and QRS is wide. This tracing may be mistaken for RVH or RBBB.

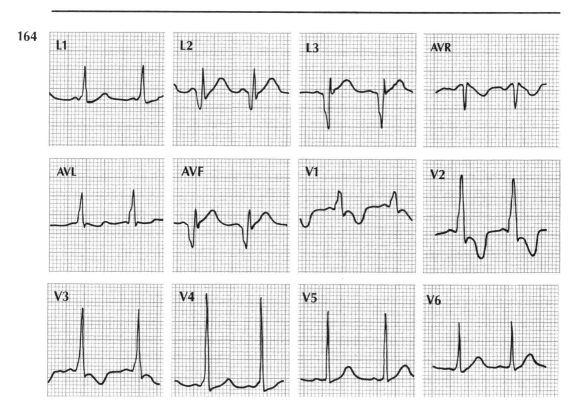

164 Wolff-Parkinson-White Syndrome:

The ECG shows the typical criteria for a Type A WPW syndrome with short PR, anterior delta wave, and wide QRS complex. This tracing may be mistaken for posteroinferior infarction, because of wide Q waves in L2, L3, AVF, and prominant R wave in lead V2.

ATRIAL AND VENTRICULAR HYPERTROPHY

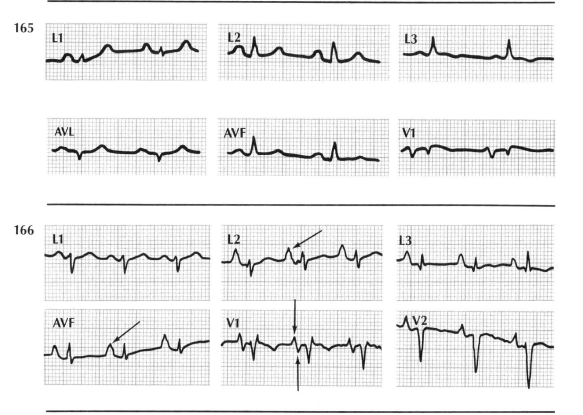

165 Left Atrial Hypertrophy:

The P wave is notched and wide in leads 1, 2, and AVF, and has a deep and wide negative phase in lead V1 with area more than one millimeter square. The patient has mitral stenosis.

166 Biatrial Hypertrophy:

The P wave is biphasic in V1. The negative phase exceeds one square millimeter, indicating LAE. The P wave in lead 2 and AVF exceeds 3 mm in amplitude indicating RAE.

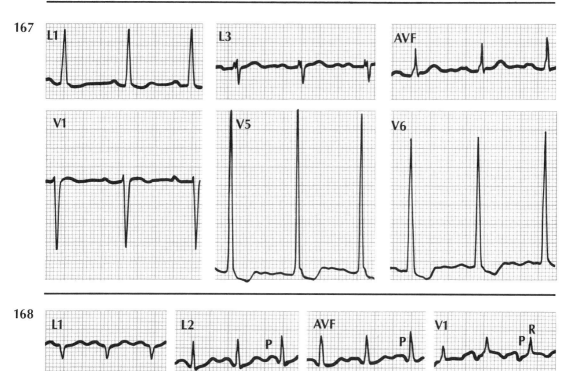

167

L1   L3   AVF

V1   V5   V6

168

L1   L2   AVF   V1

P   P   P R

167 Left Ventricular Hypertrophy:

LVH is quite evident with voltage criteria over 35 mm as the S wave in V1 and the R wave in V5 total 60 mm. The ST segment and T wave have shifted in a direction opposite to the QRS complex in leads 1, V5, and V6.

168 P Mitrale and Right Ventricular Hypertrophy:

In this tracing the P wave is more than 3 mm in duration in L1 and L2, and has a negative portion in V1 of more than 1 mm in duration and amplitude indicating LAE. The QRS axis is +120° and the R wave is prominent in V1 suggesting RVH. The above combination is seen in advanced mitral stenosis with pulmonary hypertension.

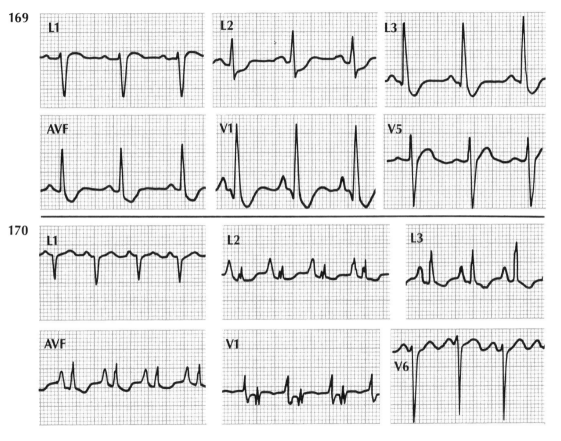

169

L1   L2   L3

AVF   V1   V5

170

L1   L2   L3

AVF   V1   V6

169 Right Ventricular and Right Atrial Enlargement:

The QRS axis is +130° and R wave is prominent in lead V1 indicating RVH. The P wave in lead V1 is peaked with 3 mm amplitude indicating RAE. The above combination is usually seen in pulmonary stenosis.

170 P Pulmonale:

Because chronic lung disease is usually the underlying cause for right atrial hypertrophy the term P pulmonale is used sometimes instead of right atrial enlargement. The P wave is tall in lead 2, 3, AVF (more than 3 mm), and in lead V1 and V2 (more than 2 mm).

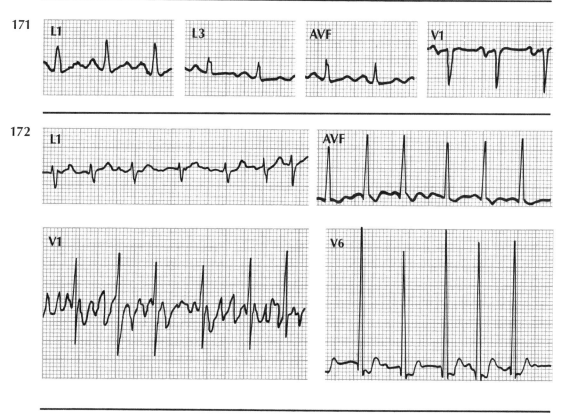

171

L1   L3   AVF   V1

172

L1   AVF

V1   V6

171 Pseudo P Mitrale:

This term is used when the ECG meets the criteria for P mitrale and the patient has no evidence of mitral disease. This tracing is from a young patient with no clinical evidence of heart disease and no reason for left atrial enlargement.

172 Biventricular Hypertrophy:

There is right axis deviation and prominant R in V1 suggesting RVH. The S wave in lead V1 and R wave in V6 equal 45, and ST is depressed in V6 indicating LVH. The underlying rhythm is atrial fibrillation. The patient has mitral stenosis and regurgitation.

SECTION VI

MYOCARDIAL INFARCTIONS AND ISCHEMIA

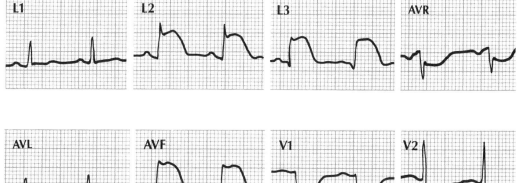
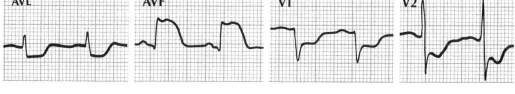
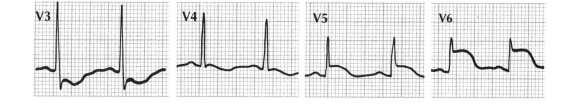

173 Acute Inferior Wall Myocardial Infarction With Reciprocal Changes:

ST segment is elevated in L2, L3, AVF, V5, and V6 which represent acute inferior lateral myocardial injury. Reciprocal ST changes are noted in leads AVL, V1, V2, and V3.

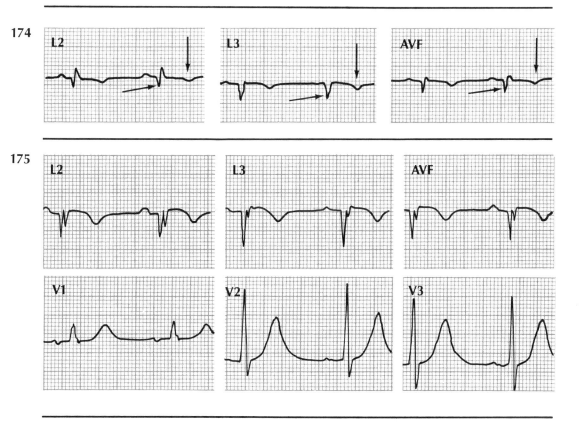

174 Old Inferior Wall Myocardial Infarction:

A significant Q wave (more than 0.03 sec) is evident in L2, L3, and AVF (→) with T inversion in these leads.

175 Old Posteroinferior Myocardial Infarction:

There is a significant Q wave and T wave inversion in L2, L3, and AVF (inferior MI). The prominent R wave in leads V1, V2, and V3 indicates involvement of the posterior wall of the left ventricle also.

176

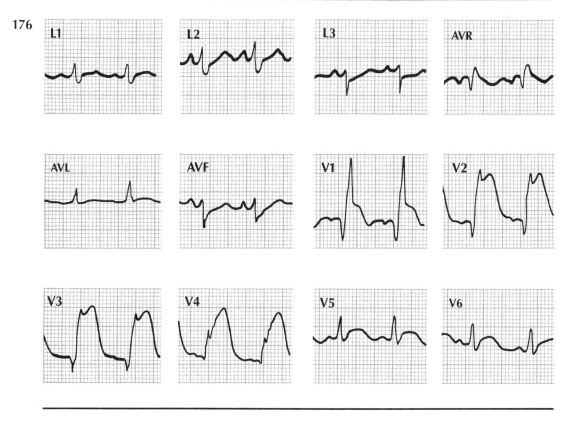

L1 L2 L3 AVR
AVL AVF V1 V2
V3 V4 V5 V6

176 Acute Extensive Anterior Myocardial Infarction:

The ST segment is strikingly elevated in the precordial leads (11 min). There is evidence of RBBB and reciprocal ST changes in L3 and AVF.

177

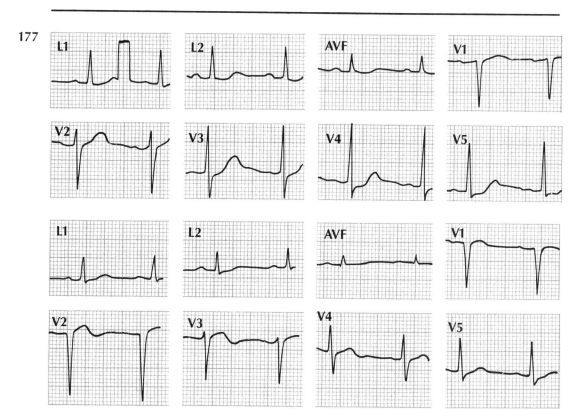

177 Anterior Wall Myocardial Infarction:

The upper ECG shows minor nonspecific ST abnormalities. The lower ECG, from the same patient, was done eleven months later, showing new QS in V1 and V2, and decreased R amplitude in V3 and V4 indicating that an anterior myocardial infarction has occurred between these two tracings.

178

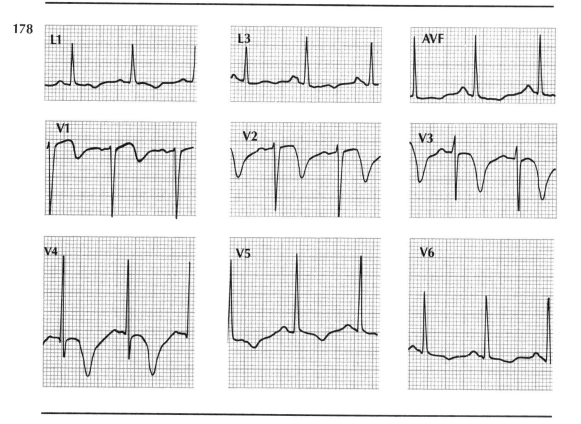

178 Subendocardial Myocardial Infarction:

The tracing shows new T wave inversion which is most prominent in V2, V3, and V4. This patient had been complaining of severe chest pain. Cardiac enzyme studies confirmed the diagnosis of a nontransmural infarction since Q waves were not present.

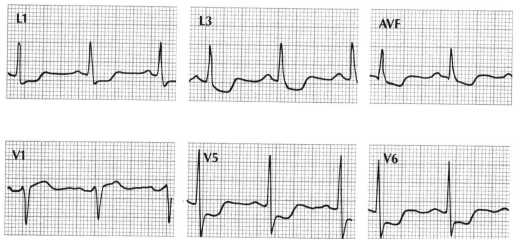

179 Ischemic ST Segment Depression:

Lead 1 reveals horizontal ST segment depression whereas L3, AVF, V5, and V6 reveals downsloping ST segments. This tracing was taken during chest pain from a 55 year old man with angina pectoris. This pattern is commonly seen with a positive treadmill stress test.

SECTION VII

SPECIAL PATTERNS

180

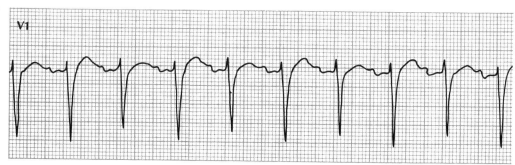

181

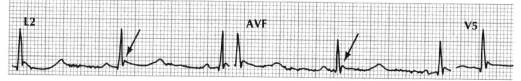

180 Electrical Alternans:

Alternating changes in QRS magnitude unrelated to respiration. If the change in QRS were associated with P wave changes, it would be called total electrical alternans. This finding may be seen in severe heart failure, pericardial effusion, or tachycardias. It can be distinguished from respiratory rhythmic variation simply by recording the ECG while the patient is holding his breath. The PR interval of .22 second indicates borderline first degree AV block.

181 Hypothermia:

J waves (arrows) are usually seen in hypothermia. Note the bradycardia (heart rate is 55), prolongation of the QT interval (.52 second), and the muscle tremor artifact, all of which are usually seen in hypothermia. This patient's temperature was below 90 degrees F.

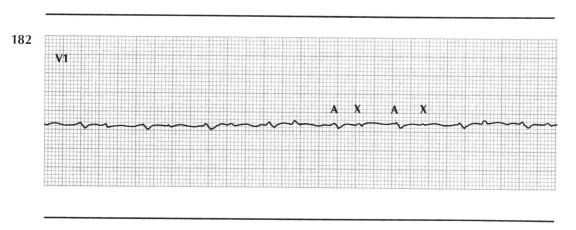

182

V1

A X A X

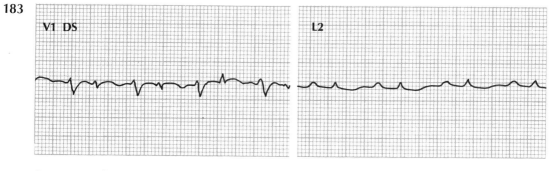

183

V1 DS

L2

Strips 182 and 183 are from the same patient.

182 Emphysema:

This patient has sinus rhythm, first degree AV block, and low voltage. The QRS complex is smaller than the P wave. A denotes the P wave, and X denotes the QRS complex. The PR interval is .28 second. This patient has severe, chronic, obstructive pulmonary disease.

Strips 182 and 183 are from the same patient.

183 Emphysema:

Same patient as strip 182. Lead V1 is now recorded in double standard (DS). The QRS is now more easily visualized. First degree AV block is present (PR .28). The P wave in V1 shows left atrial enlargement, which gives it the appearance of a QRS complex.

184

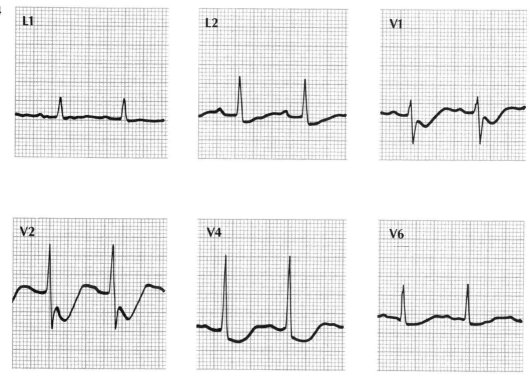

184 Hypokalemia:

The QU segment is markedly prolonged (0.56 sec) in V2. Serum potassium was 2 mEq/L.

185

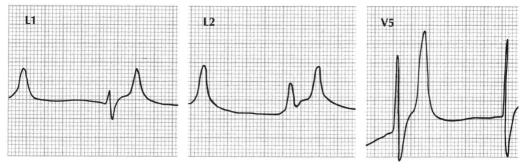

186

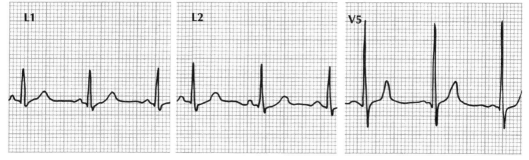

Strips 185 and 186 are from the same patient.

185 Hyperkalemia:

This strip shows the P-QRS-T changes of advanced hyperkalemia. The P waves are flat, the QRS duration is long, and the T wave is peaked. Serum potassium of this patient was 9 mEq-/liter.

Strips 185 and 186 are from the same patient.

186 Sinus Rhythm:

This rhythm strip was obtained from the same patient (strip 185) before he developed hyperkalemia.

187

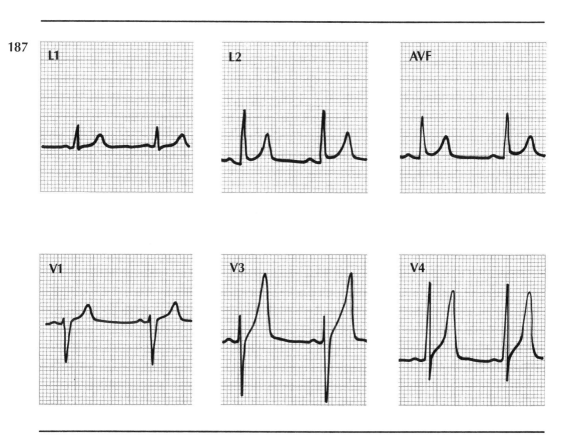

187 Early Repolarization:

The J point and ST segment are slightly elevated in L2, AVF, V3, and V4, indicating early repolarization. The T wave is peaked in V3 and V4. This phenomena is a normal variation.

188

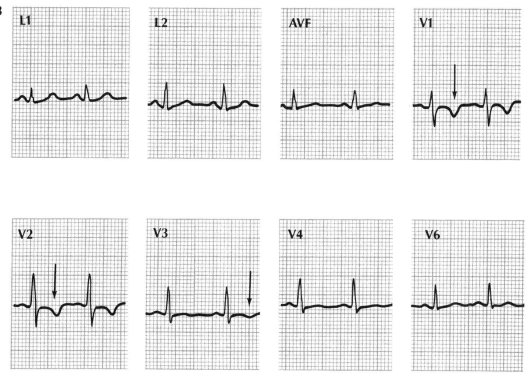

188 Juvenile T Wave:

The T wave is inverted in lead V1, V2, and V3. This ECG is from a 12 year old girl. This pattern may be seen normally in women, young children, and blacks.

189

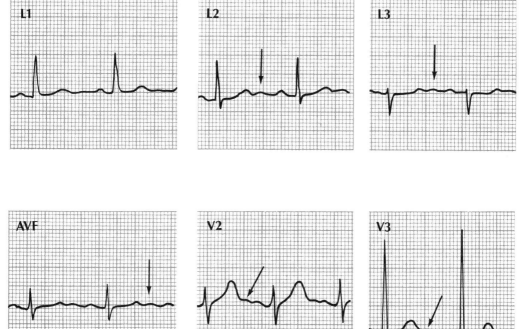

189 Normal U Wave:

A normal U wave (↓) should be a half or less of the T wave amplitude and upright.

190

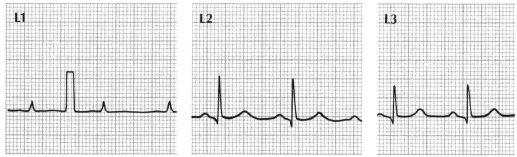

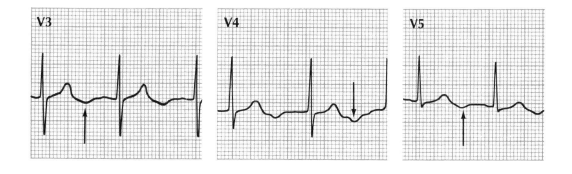

190 Negative U Wave:

The U wave is inverted in lead V3, V4, and V5 (↑↓). U wave inversion is usually associated with organic heart disease.

191

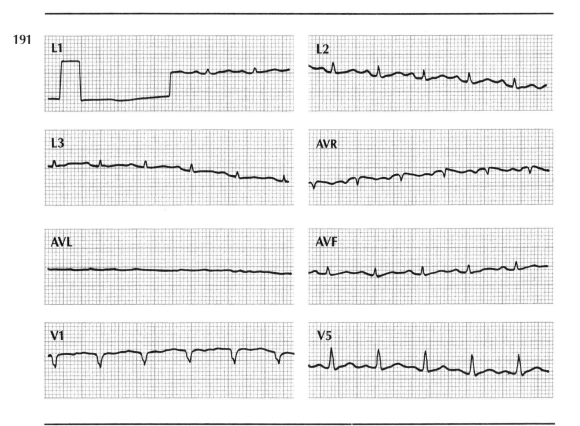

191 Low Voltage and Pericardial Effusion:

The ECG is from a 20 year old man with a large pericardial effusion proved by echocardiography. Note that the sum of the amplitude of QRS complexes of any two limb leads does not exceed 10 mm.

192

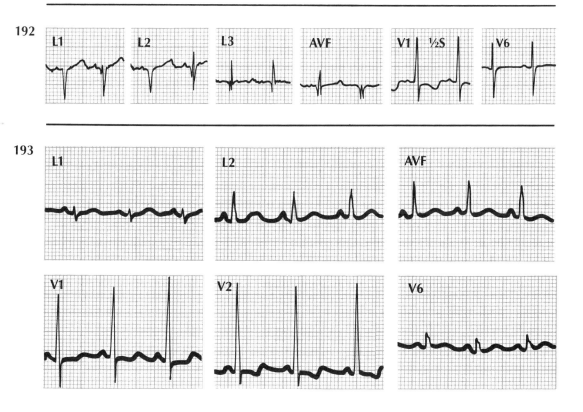

193

192 Normal Newborn:

The QRS axis is about +140° and the R wave is larger than S wave in lead V1. These findings are normal for the newborn but they represent right ventricular hypertrophy in the adult.

193 Tetralogy of Fallot:

This ECG is from a five year old boy, and shows right ventricular hypertrophy. Tetralogy of Fallot was confirmed by cardiac catheterization.

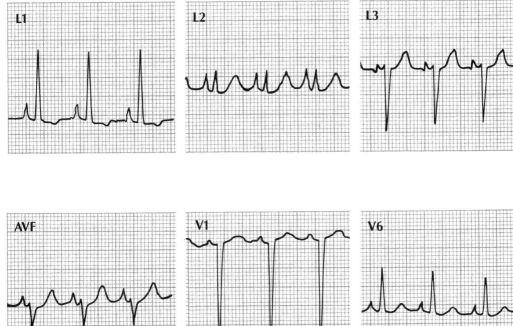

194 Tricuspid Atresia:

Left axis deviation (QRS axis is -20°), right atrial enlargement, and voltage criteria for left ventricular hypertrophy are the basic criteria for tricuspid atresia. The ECG is from a six year old boy. The term P congenitale is sometimes used if the criteria for right atrial enlargement exists in a patient with congenital heart disease.

195

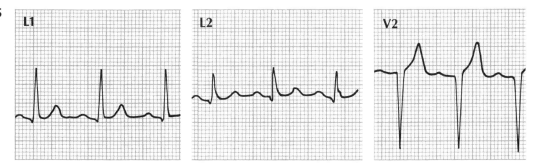

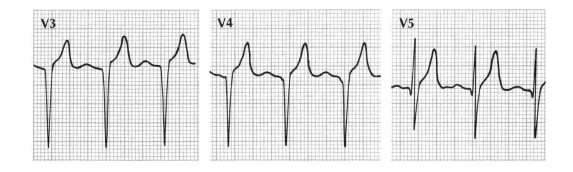

195 Idiopathic Hypertrophic Subaortic Stenosis:

The ECG is from a 39 year old man who never had a heart attack. Auscultation revealed a systolic murmur which increased with Valsalva maneuver. The ECG shows QS in V2, V3, and V4, simulating an anterior infarction. The echocardiogram demonstrated a thick intraventricular septum.

196

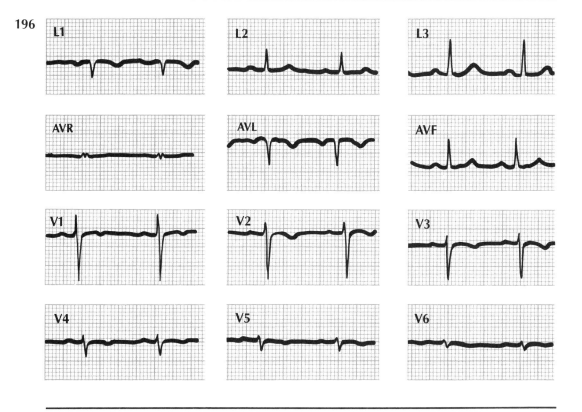

196 Dextrocardia:

Lead 1 is inverted and there is a poor R progression from V1 to V6. Reversal of arm lead electrodes is associated with normal progression of R in the chest leads. Whenever the P wave in lead I is inverted the ECG should be repeated, since arm lead reversal occurs more commonly than dextrocardia.

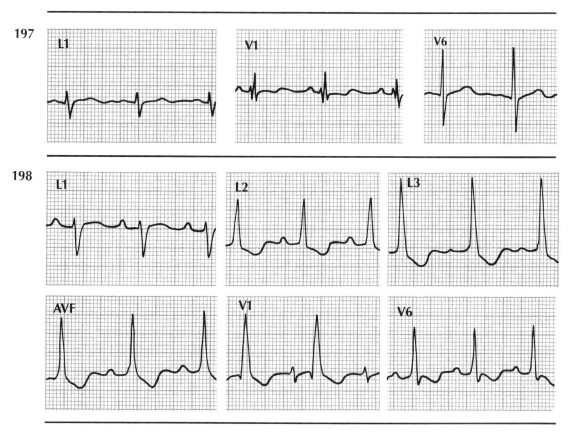

197

L1   V1   V6

198

L1   L2   L3

AVF   V1   V6

197 Atrial Septal Defect:

Atrial septal defect should be suspected in every case of IRBBB. This tracing is from a young man with a heart murmur since birth.

198 Eisenmenger Syndrome:

The ECG is from a 12 year old boy with atrial septal defect and significant pulmonary hypertension proven by cardiac catheterization. Eisenmenger syndrome implies pulmonary hypertension with reversal of the left to right shunt at atrial, ventricular, or pulmonary artery level. This tracing shows RVH and first degree AV block. The biatrial hypertrophy (V1) suggests that the underlying cardiac lesion is atrial septal defect.

INDEX

(Note: Numeric references refer to strip numbers. Those in parentheses
refer to page numbers.)

Aberrant conduction and aberrancy:
  Ashman phenomenon, 118
  atrial escape, 9
  atrial fibrillation, 119
  features of, 121
  premature atrial complexes, 8, 42, 109, 114
  right bundle branch block, 116
  supraventricular tachycardia, 115, 125
Accelerated idioventricular rhythm:
  atrial flutter with complete heart block, 51
  fusion complexes, 84
  heart rates, (8)
  see also Idioventricular rhythm
Accelerated junctional rhythm:
  atrial fibrillation, 29
  heart rates, (8)
  see also Junctional rhythm
Accessory bundle, 151
Acute extensive anterior myocardial infarction,
      176
Acute inferior wall myocardial infarction, 173
Alternans, see Electrical alternans
Alternating bundle branch block, 152

Angina pectoris, 179
Antegrade conduction, 149
Anterior hemiblock, see Left anterior hemiblock
Anterior wall myocardial infarction, 177
Arrhythmias:
  heart rates and, (8)
  see also entries under names of specific
      arrhythmias
Ashman phenomenon:
  aberrant conduction, 119, 121
  features of, 118
  premature ventricular complex, 65
  Wolff-Parkinson-White syndrome
      differentiated from, 122
Atresia (tricuspid), 194
Atrial bigeminy:
  premature atrial complexes with, and
      trigemy and quadrigeminy, 40
  sinus arrest differentiated from, 106
  see also Ventricular bigeminy
Atrial complex (interpolated premature), 46
Atrial depolarization, 60
Atrial enlargement, see Left atrial hypertrophy;

Atrial enlargement *(continued) see* Right atrial
   hypertrophy
Atrial escape:
  blocked premature atrial complex, 41
  features of, 9
  ventricular group complexes, 62
Atrial fibrillation:
  aberrant conduction, 118, 119, 121, 125
  accelerated junctional rhythm, 29
  atrial flutter contrasted, 51
  biventricular hypertrophy, 172
  conversion of sinus rhythm to, 25
  conversion to sinus rhythm of, 26
  features of, 22
  fine atrial fibrillation, 24, 36
  heart rates, (8)
  junctional escape rhythm and premature
       ventricular complexes, 39
  junctional rhythm, 38
  left bundle branch block, 113
  pacemaker (R-triggered), 89
  premature ventricular complex, 65
  regular rhythm contrasted, 37
  right bundle branch block, 124
  third degree AV block, 139
  ventricular bigeminy, 23
  Wolff-Parkinson-White syndrome, 122
Atrial flutter:

Atrial flutter: *(continued)*
  complete heart block and accelerated
       idioventricular rhythm, 51
  heart rates, (8)
  junctional tachycardia and complete AV
       dissociation, 21
  premature ventricular complex, 65
  sinus tachycardia, 4
  2:1 AV block, 18, 19, 20
  2:1 AV conduction present, carotid massage
       effect, 15
  Wenckebach AV block (8:3), 17
Atrial hypertrophy, *see* Left atrial hypertrophy;
       Right atrial hypertrophy
Atrial pacemaker, 93
Atrial premature complexes, *see* Premature
       atrial complexes
Atrial quadrigeminy, *see* Quadrigeminy
Atrial septal defect:
  Eisenmenger syndrome, 198
  incomplete right bundle branch block, 197
Atrial tachycardia:
  atrial flutter differentiated from, 19
  first degree AV block present, 12
  heart rates, (8)
  multifocal, 34
  paroxysmal, 11
  third degree AV block with, 140

Atrial tachycardia: *(continued)*

    2:1 AV block and, 13, 14, 44
    Wenckebach AV block and, 110
Atrioventricular block, *see* First degree AV
       block; Second degree AV block; Third
       degree AV block; *entries under names of*
       specific heart blocks
Atrioventricular dissociation, 145, 149
Atrioventricular node:
  blocked premature atrial complex, 148
  concealed conduction, 120
  interpolated premature ventricular complex
      with concealed conduction, 69
  right bundle branch block and first degree AV
      block, 154
  sinus block, 104
  ventricular bigeminy, 54
Axis determination, (4)

Biatrial hypertrophy:
  Eisenmenger syndrome, 198
  left atrial hypertrophy, 166
Bidirectional ventricular tachycardia, 74
Bifascicular block, 155
Bigeminy, *see* Atrial bigeminy; Ventricular
    bigeminy
Bilateral bundle branch block, 158

Bipolar right ventricular pacemaker, 96
Biventricular hypertrophy, 172. *See also* Left
      ventricular hypertrophy; Right ventricular
      hypertrophy
Blocked antegrade/retrograde conduction, 64
Blocked premature atrial complexes:
  atrial escape, 41
  features of, 133, 146, 148
  see also Premature atrial complexes
Bradycardia, 181. *see also* Sinus bradycardia
Bradycardia-tachycardia syndrome, 7
Bundle branch block:
  atrial fibrillation and accelerated junctional
      rhythm, 29
  ventricular escape complex, 97
  see also Intermittent right bundle branch
      block; Left bundle branch block; Right
      bundle branch block.
Bundle of His:
  right bundle branch block and first degree AV
      block, 154
  right bundle branch block and first degree AV
      block, and left anterior hemiblock, 156,
      157
  second degree AV block, 132
  trifascicular block/monofascicular block
      differentiated from, 160, 161

Cardiac arrest, 78
Cardiac enzyme studies, 178
Carotid massage:
    atrial flutter and, with 2:1 AV conduction, 15
    atrial tachycardia with Wenckebach AV block, 110
    first degree AV block, 128
    paroxysmal atrial tachycardia converted to sinus rhythm by, 11
    supraventricular tachycardia with aberrancy, 115
    supraventricular versus ventricular tachycardia, 73
Carotid sinus pressure:
    atrial tachycardia with 2:1 AV block, 44
    sinus tachycardia, 6
Chronic lung disease, 170. See also Emphysema
Complete AV block, see Third degree AV block
Complete AV dissociation, 21
Complete heart block, see Third degree AV block
Concealed conduction:
    atrial flutter with 2:1 AV block, 18
    features of, 120
    interpolated premature junctional complexes, 45
    interpolated premature ventricular complexes, 67, 69, 82

Concealed conduction: (continued)
    ventricular bigeminy, 83
Conduction, see Aberrant conduction and aberrancy; Concealed conduction
Congenital disorders:
    cataracts, blocked premature atrial complexes, 146
    paroxysmal ventricular tachycardia due to prolongation of QT interval, 100
    tricuspid atresia, 194
Coronary nodal rhythm, 49
Coronary sinus rhythm, see Sinus rhythm
Coronary sinus tachycardia, see Sinus tachycardia
Coupling interval:
    Ashman phenomenon, 118
    premature ventricular complex, 64
    ventricular parasystole, 81

DC shock, 73
Demand pacemaker:
    malfunctioning, 92
    pacemaker-induced complexes, 91
    premature ventricular complex, 87, 90
    see also Pacemaker
Dextrocardia, 196
Digitalis toxicity:
    double tachycardia, 21
    third degree AV block, 139

Early repolarization, 187
Ectopic atrial focus, 6
Eisenmenger syndrome, 198
Electrical alternans:
 respiratory rhythmic variation differentiated
  from, 190
 supraventricular tachycardia with, 43
Emphysema, 182, 183
End-diastolic premature ventricular complex, 60
Enzyme studies, 178
Escape, *see* Atrial escape; Junctional escape;
  Sinus escape; Ventricular escape
Exercise-induced ventricular tachycardia, 72
Extrasystole, 66

Fibrillation, *see* Atrial fibrillation; Ventricular
  fibrillation
Fine atrial fibrillation, 24
 features, 36
 see also Atrial fibrillation
First degree AV block:
 alternating bundle branch block, 152
 atrial tachycardia with, 12
 bradycardia-tachycardia syndrome, 7
 carotid massage, 128
 clarification of, 127
 concealed conduction, 120
 demand pacemaker, 90
 Eisenmenger syndrome, 198

First degree AV block: *(continued)*

 electrical alternans, 180
 emphysema, 182, 183
 features of, 103
 inferior myocardial infarction, posterior
  hemiblock and, 160
 interpolated premature ventricular complex
  with concealed conduction, 69
 junctional rhythm, 126
 left anterior hemiblock, 161
 right bundle branch block, 154
 right bundle branch block and left anterior
  hemiblock, 156, 157
 sinus block, 104, 105
 sinus bradycardia with incomplete AV
  dissociation, 149
 sinus bradycardia with junctional escape, 48
 sinus tachycardia with, 111, 112
 third degree AV block differentiated from,
  143
 ventricular bigeminy with concealed
  conduction, 83
 ventricular trigeminy differentiated from,
  57
 see also Second degree AV block; Third
  degree AV block; *entries under names
  of specific heart blocks*
Fixed rate pacemaker, 88
Fusion complexes, 84

Heart block, *see* First degree AV block; Second degree AV block; Third degree AV block; *entries under names of specific heart blocks*

Heart rate:
  basic arrhythmias and, (8)
  determination table for, (3)
  sinus tachycardia, 4

Hemiblock, *see* Left anterior hemiblock; Left posterior hemiblock; Posterior hemiblock

Hexaxial reference system, (5)

His studies, *see* Bundle of His

Hyperkalemia, 185

Hypertrophy, *see* Left atrial hypertrophy; Left ventricular hypertrophy; Right atrial hypertrophy; Right ventricular hypertrophy

Hypokalemia:
  features of, 184
  paroxysmal ventricular tachycardia due to prolongation of QT interval, 100

Hypothermia, 181

Idiopathic hypertrophic subaortic stenosis, 195

Idioventricular rhythm:
  heart rates, (8)
  ventricular escape, 86
  ventricular/junctional escape, 98

Idioventricular rhythm (accelerated):
  atrial flutter with complete heart block, 51
  fusion complexes, 84
  heart rates, (8)

Incomplete AV dissociation, 149

Incomplete right bundle branch block, 97

Inferior myocardial infarction, 160

Inferolateral myocardial infarction, *see* Inferior myocardial infarction

Intermittent left bundle branch block:
  bilateral bundle branch block, 158
  features of, 135, 136
  premature ventricular complexes, 162
  see also Bundle branch block; Left bundle branch block

Intermittent right bundle branch block:
  atrial septal defect, 197
  bilateral bundle branch block, 158
  end-diastolic premature ventricular complex contrasted, 117
  normal variant, 153
  see also Bundle branch block; Right bundle branch block

Incomplete right bundle branch block, 153

Intermittent Wolff-Parkinson-White syndrome, 150. *See also* Wolff-Parkinson-White syndrome

Interpolated premature atrial complex, 46

Interpolated premature junctional complex, 45

Interpolated premature ventricular complex:
  concealed conduction, 67, 69, 82
  features of, 66
Ischemic ST segment depression, 179
Isoproterenol, 144

Junctional complexes:
  interpolated premature, 45
  third degree AV block, 138
Junctional escape:
  atrial fibrillation with, and premature
      ventricular complexes, 39
  features of, 47
  sinus bradycardia with, 48
  ventricular escape complex and, 98
Junctional node inertia, 7
Junctional premature complexes, see Premature
      junctional complexes
Junctional rhythm:
  accelerated, atrial fibrillation and, 29
  atrial fibrillation differentiated from, 37
  atrial fibrillation with, 38
  coronary sinus rhythm, 50
  features of, 28
  first degree AV block and, 126, 128
  heart rates, (8)
  multiform premature ventricular complexes,
      101

Junctional rhythm: (Continued)
  sinus tachycardia with AV dissociation, 145
  third degree AV block, 138
  ventricular bigeminy and, 83
Junctional tachycardia:
  artrial flutter with, and complete AV
      dissociation, 21
  heart rates, (8)
  midnodal, 30
  sinus tachycardia with first degree AV block,
      111
  supraventricular tachycardia, 32
Juvenile T wave, 188
J wave, 181

Left anterior hemiblock:
  first degree AV block, 161
  right bundle branch block, 155
  right bundle branch block and first degree AV
      block, 156, 157
Left atrial hypertrophy:
  bilateral hypertrophy, 166
  emphysema, 183
  features of, 165
  pseudo P mitrate, 171
Left atrial rhythm, 50
Left bundle branch block:

Left bandle branch block: *(continued)*

    alternating bundle branch block, 152
    atrial fibrillation, 113
    left posterior hemiblock, 159
    pacemaker and, 94
    premature ventricular complex (multi-form),
        53
Left bundle branch block (intermittent):
    bilateral bundle branch block, 158
    features of, 135, 136
    premature ventricular complexes, 162
Left posterior hemiblock, 159
Left ventricular hypertrophy:
    biventricular hypertrophy, 172
    features of, 167
    right atrial hypertrophy and, 169
    tricuspid atresia, 194
LGL syndrome, *see* Lown-Ganong-Levine
       syndrome
Lidocaine, 85
Lown-Ganong-Levine syndrome, 49
Low voltage, 191
Lung disease (chronic), 170. *See also*
       Emphysema

Malignant pericardial effusion, 43
Midnodal accelerated junctional rhythm, *see*
       Accelerated junctional rhythm
Midnodal junctional tachycardia, 30

Mitral stenosis:
    biventricular hypertrophy, 172
    left atrial hypertrophy, 165
    right ventricular hypertrophy and P mitrale,
       168
Mobitz, *see* Second degree AV block, Mobitz
Monofascicular block:
    determination of, 154
    trifascicular block differentiated from, 160,
       161
Multifocal atrial tachycardia:
    features of, 34
    heart rates, (8)
Multiform premature ventricular complex, 53,
       59, 101
Murmur:
    atrial septal defect, 197
    systolic murmur, 194
Muscle tremor artifact:
    hypothermia, 181
    second degree AV block, 137
Myocardial infarction:
    acute extensive anterior, 176
    acute inferior wall, 173
    anterior wall, 177
    inferior, 160
    old inferior wall, 174
    old posteroinferior, 175
    subendocardial, 178
    Type I, (6)

Myocardial infarchon: *(continued)*

Type II, (7)
Myocarditis, 145

Neonate, 192. *See also* Pediatrics
Nodal rhythm, (8)

Old inferior wall myocardial infarction, 174
Old posteroinferior myocardial infarction, 175

Pacemaker:
   atrial, 93
   bipolar right ventricular, 96
   demand pacemaker, 87, 90, 91, 92
   fixed rate pacemaker, 88
   idioventricular rhythm, 86
   myocarditis, 145
   R-triggered pacemaker, 89
   sinus arrest, 107
   unipolar left ventricular, 95
   unipolar right ventricular, 94
   see also Wandering pacemaker
Pairing, 56
Parasystolic focus:
   premature ventricular complex, 64
   ventricular parasystole, 80, 81
Paroxysmal atrial tachycardia:
   conversion to sinus rhythm by carotid
      massage, 11

Paroxysmal atrial tachycardia: *(continued)*

first degree AV block present, 12
Paroxysmal tachycardia, 49
Paroxysmal ventricular tachycardia, 100
P congenitale, 194
Pediatrics:
   Eisenmenger syndrome, 198
   juvenile T wave, 188
   newborn (normal), 192
   tetralogy of Fallot, 193
   tricuspid atresis, 194
Pericardial effusion:
   electrical alternans, 43
   low voltage, 191
Pharmacology:
   isoproterenol, 144
   lidocaine, 85
   procainamide, 101
   quinidine, 101
   ventricular tachycardia, exercise-induced, 72
P mitrale:
   pseudo P mitrale, 171
   right ventricular hypertrophy, 168
Posterior hemiblock:
   inferior myocardial infarction, 160
   left posterior hemiblock, 159
   see also Left anterior hemiblock;
Posteroinferior infarction, 164
Postextrasystolic pause, 162

Post-premature ventricular complex, 68
Potassium, see Hyperkalemia; Hypokalemia
P pulmonale, 170. See also Right atrial
    hypertrophy
Precordial thump, 71
Premature atrial complexes:
  aberrancy, 42, 109
  atrial escape, 9
  bigeminy, trigeminy, quadrigeminy, 40
  blocked, atrial escape, 41
  blocked, features of, 133, 146, 148
  end-diastolic PVC differentiated from, 60
  features of, 8
  first degree AV block, 103
  interpolated, 46
  premature ventricular complexes and, 52
  sinus rhythm converted to atrial fibrillation,
    25
  variable aberrancy and, 114
Premature atrial complexes (interpolated), 46
Premature junctional complexes:
  end-diastolic premature ventricular
    complexes, 60
  features of, 27
  interpolated, 45
Premature ventricular complexes:
  atrial escape and blocked premature atrial
    complex, 41
  atrial fibrillation and, 65

Premature ventricular complexes: (continued)

  atrial fibrillation with junctional escape
    rhythm, 39
  atrial fibrillation with ventricular bigeminy, 23
  bradycardia-tachycardia syndrome, 7
  concealed conduction, 120
  different coupling intervals, 64
  end-diastolic, 60
  features of, 52, 58, 99
  first degree AV block, 103
  group complexes, 62
  intermittent right bundle branch block
    contrasted, 117
  left bundle branch block and, 162
  pacemaker (demand), 87, 90
  pacemaker (fixed rate), 88
  pairing and, 56
  premature atrial complexes with aberrancy
    contrasted, 109
  R on T phenomenon, 61
  T wave changes after, 68
  ventricular bigeminy and, 54, 57
  ventricular quadrigeminy and, 63
  ventricular tachycardia and, 75
  ventricular trigeminy and, 55
Premature ventricular complexes (interpolated):
  concealed conduction and, 67, 69, 82
  features of, 66

Premature ventricular complexes (multiform), 53, 59, 101
Procainamide, 101
Pseudo P mitrale, 171
Pulmonary disease, see Emphysema
Pulmonary hypertension:
  Eisenmenger syndrome, 198
  right ventricular hypertrophy and P mitrale, 168
Pulmonary stenosis, 169

QRS axis determination, (4)
Quadrigeminy:
  atrial premature complexes with, 40
  ventricular, 63
Quinidine:
  atrial flutter and, 20
  paroxysmal ventricular tachycardia due to prolongation of QT interval, 100
  premature ventricular complexes, 101

Race differences, 188
Reciprocal changes, 173
Regurgitation, 172
Repolarization (early), 187
Respiration:
  sinus arrhythmia, 1, 2, 3
  sinus block, 105
Respiratory rhythmic variation:

Respiratory rhythmic variation: (continued)
  electrical alternans differentiated from, 180
  features of, 2
Right atrial hypertrophy:
  P pulmonale, 170
  right ventricular hypertrophy and, 169
  tricuspid atresia, 194
  see also Left atrial hypertrophy; Left ventricular hypertrophy; Right ventricular hypertrophy
Right bundle branch block:
  aberrant conduction, 116
  alternating bundle branch block, 152
  Ashman phenomenon, 118
  atrial flutter, 16
  features of, 124
  first degree AV block 154
  first degree AV block and left anterior hemiblock, 156, 157
  incomplete, 153
  interpolated premature junctional complexes with, 45
  left anterior hemiblock and, 155
  myocardial infarction, 176
  pacemaker and, 95
  premature atrial complexes with aberrancy, 109
  premature atrial complexes with variable

Right bundle branch block: *(continued)*

      aberrancy, 114
   supraventricular versus ventricular
      tachycardia, 73
   Wolff-Parkinson-White syndrome
      differentiated from, 163
   see also Bundle branch block; Intermittent
      right bundle branch block; Left bundle
      branch block
Right ventricular hypertrophy:
   biventricular hypertrophy, 172
   Eisenmenger syndrome, 198
   P mitrale and, 168
   right atrial hypertrophy and, 169
   sinus tachycardia and, 6
   tetralogy of Fallot, 193
   Wolff-Parkinson-White syndrome
      differentiated from, 163
   see also Left ventricular hypertrophy
R on T phenomenon, 61

Second degree AV block:
   bundle of His recordings, 132
   intermittent left bundle branch block, 135,
      136
   Mobitz Type I, 4:3 block, 130
   Mobitz Type I, Mobitz Type II differentiated
      from, 131, 132

Second degree AV block: *(continued)*

   Mobitz Type I, Wenckebach, 129
   Mobitz Type II, Mobitz Type I differentiated
      from, 131, 132
   muscle tremor artifact and, 137
   premature atrial complexes differentiated
      from, 133
   second degree sinus block contrasted, 108
   sinus bradycardia differentiated from, 147
   third degree AV block differentiated from,
      142
Second degree sinus block:
   Type I (Wenckebach), 108
   see also Sinus block
Sex differences, 188
Sick sinus syndrome:
   bradycardia-tachycardia syndrome, 7
   sinus arrest, 107
   sinus block, 104
Sinoatrial node, 10
Sinus arrest:
   bradycardia-tachycardia syndrome, 7
   cardiac arrest, 78
   sick sinus syndrome, 107
   sinus bradycardia differentiated from, 106
Sinus arrhythmia:
   features of, 1
   heart rates, (8)

Sinus arrhythmia: *(continued)*

respiratory cycle and, 3, 105
sinus arrest, 107
sinus bradycardia with, 5
U waves, 134
ventriculophasic sinus arrhythmia, 141, 142

Sinus block:
sick sinus syndrome, 104
see also Second degree sinus block

Sinus bradycardia:
heart rates, (8)
incomplete AV dissociation, 149
junctional escape and, 48
second degree AV block differentiated from, 147
sinus arrest differentiated from, 106
sinus arrhythmia with, 5
third degree AV block differentiated from, 143
U waves, 134

Sinus complex:
post-premature ventricular complex T wave changes, 68
ventricular trigeminy, 55

Sinus escape complex, 71

Sinus rhythm:
atrial escape and, 41
atrial fibrillation differentiated from, 37, 38

Sinus rhythm: *(continued)*

atrial tachycardia, 110
concealed conduction, 120
conversion of atrial fibrillation to, 26
conversion to atrial fibrillation of, 25
emphysema, 182
features of, 50
fusion complexes, 84
heart rates, (8)
hyperkalemia and, 186
intermittent left bundle branch block and premature ventricular complexes, 162
lidocaine and, 85
paroxysmal atrial tachycardia converted to, by carotid massage, 11
right bundle branch block and, 124
spontaneous conversion to, atrial tachycardia, 12
supraventricular tachycardia converted to, 10, 32
ventricular bigeminy and, 83
ventricular tachycardia with spontaneous conversion to, 70

Sinus tachycardia:
atrial flutter differentiated from, 15, 19
atrial tachycardia differentiated, 14
atrial tachycardia with Wenckebach AV block, 110

Index

261

Sinus tachycardia: *(continued)*
    atrioventricular dissociation and, 145
    carotid sinus pressure and, 6
    features of, 31
    first degree AV block and, 111, 112
    heart rates, (8)
    paroxysmal atrial tachycardia differentiated
        from, 11
Standstill, *see* Ventricular standstill
ST segment depression (ischemic), 179
Subaortic stenosis (idiopathic hypertrophic),
    195
Subendocardial myocardial infarction, 178
Supraventricular tachycardia:
    aberrancy and, 115, 125
    conversion to sinus rhythm by Valsalva
        maneuver, 10
    electrical alternans and, 43
    junctional tachycardia, 32
    lidocaine and, 85
    ventricular tachycardia versus, 73
    see also Atrial tachycardia; Junctional
        tachycardia; Ventricular tachycardia
Systolic murmur, 194

Tachycardia, *see entries under specific*
    tachycardias
Tetralogy of Fallot, 193

Third degree AV block:
    atrial fibrillation and, 139
    atrial flutter with, and accelerated
        idioventricular rhythm, 51
    atrial tachycardia and, 140
    features of, 138
    isoproterenol and, 144
    right bundle branch block, first degree AV
        block, left anterior hemiblock and, 157
    second degree AV block differentiated from,
        142
    sinus bradycardia differentiated from, 143
    ventriculophasic sinus arrhythmia and, 141,
        142
    see also First degree AV block; Second
        degree AV block; *entries under names*
        specific heart blocks
Torsades de pointes:
    features of, 102
    heart rates and, (8)
    premature ventricular complexes (multi-form)
        and, 101
Tricuspid atresia, 194
Trifascicular block:
    alternating bundle branch block, 152
    bilateral bundle branch block, 158
    monofascicular block differentiated from,
        160, 161

Trifascicular block: *(continued)*

    right bundle branch block, first degree AV
        block, 154
    right bundle branch block, first degree AV
        block, and left anterior hemiblock, 156,
        157

Trigeminy:
  atrial flutter with, and trigeminal rhythm, 16
  atrial premature complexes with, and
      bigeminy and quadrigeminy, 40
  ventricular trigeminy, 55

T wave, 68
T wave (juvenile), 188

2:1 AV block:
  atrial flutter with, 18, 19, 20
  atrial tachycardia, 13, 14, 44
  blocked premature atrial complexes
      differentiated from, 146
  intermittent left bundle branch block, 135
  muscle tremor artifact and, 137
  sinus tachycardia and, 4

2:1 AV conduction, 15

Unipolar left ventricular pacemaker, 95
Unipolar right ventricular pacemaker, 94

U wave:
  negative, 190
  normal, 189

U wave: *(continued)*

  sinus bradycardia, 134

Vagus nerve, 115

Valsalva maneuver:
  supraventricular tachycardia converted to
      sinus rhythm by, 10
  systolic murmur, 195

Variable aberrancy, *see* Aberrant conduction
    and aberrancy

Ventricular bigeminy:
  atrial fibrillation with, 23
  concealed conduction and, 83
  first degree AV block, 103
  first degree AV block differentiated from, 57
  premature ventricular complex and, 54
  see also Atrial bigeminy

Ventricular escape:
  features of, 97
  idioventricular rhythm, 86
  junctional escape complex and, 98
  sinus tachycardia with AV dissociation, 145
  supraventricular tachycardia, 10

Ventricular fibrillation:
  cardiac arrest, 78
  complete distortion/irregularity of all
      complexes, 76
  heart rates and, (8)

Ventricular fibrillation: *(continued)*

R on T phenomenon, 61
smaller amplitude, 77
Ventricular flutter:
features of, 79
heart rates and, (8)
Ventricular group complexes, 62
Ventricular hypertrophy, *see* Left ventricular
hypertrophy; Right ventricular
hypertrophy
Ventricular parasystole:
coupling intervals, 81
fusion complexes, 80
heart rates and, (8)
Ventricular premature complexes, *see*
Premature ventricular complexes
Ventricular quadrigeminy, 63
Ventricular standstill:
cardiac arrest, 78
sinus tachycardia with AV dissociation, 145
Ventricular tachycardia:
aberrant conduction, 125
atrial fibrillation and left bundle branch block
contrasted, 113
bidirectional, 74
bradycardia-tachycardia syndrome, 7
conversion by precordial thump, 71

Ventricular tachycardia: *(continued)*

exercise-induced, 72
heart rates and, (8)
lidocaine and, 85
paroxysmal, 100
premature ventricular complexes and, 75
R on T phenomenon, 61
spontaneous conversion to sinus rhythm, 70
supraventricular tachycardia versus, 73
supraventricular tachycardia with aberrancy
contrasted, 115
torsades de pointes, 101, 102
ventricular flutter compared, 79
ventricular group complexes, 62
Ventricular tachycardia (paroxysmal), 100
Ventricular trigeminy:
features of, 55
see also Trigeminy
Ventriculophasic sinus arrhythmia, 141, 142

Wandering pacemaker:
heart rates, (8)
sinus node, junctional tissue, 35
sinus node, junctional tissue, and various
atrial locations, 33
Wenckebach AV block:
atrial flutter with, 17

Wenckebach AV block: *(continued)*

    atrial flutter with, and trigeminal rhythm, 16
    atrial tachycardia with, 110
    complete AV block and, 144
    4:3 block, 130
    Mobitz I and II differentiated, 131, 132
    second degree AV block, Mobitz Type I, 129
    see also Second degree sinus block
Wolff-Parkinson-White syndrome:
    Ashman phenomenon distinguished from,
        122
    differentiation of, 163
    features of, 123, 151
    intermittent, 150
    posteroinferior infarction differentiated from,
        164